Pituitary Disorders

Editors

ANAT BEN-SHLOMO
MARIA FLESERIU

ENDOCRINOLOGY AND METABOLISM CLINICS OF NORTH AMERICA

www.endo.theclinics.com

Consulting Editor
DEREK LeROITH

March 2015 • Volume 44 • Number 1

ELSEVIER

1600 John F. Kennedy Boulevard ● Suite 1800 ● Philadelphia, Pennsylvania, 19103-2899

http://www.theclinics.com

ENDOCRINOLOGY AND METABOLISM CLINICS OF NORTH AMERICA Volume 44, Number 1
March 2015 ISSN 0889-8529, ISBN 13: 978-0-323-35654-1

Editor: Jessica McCool
Developmental Editor: Meredith Clinton

Endocrinology and Metabolism Clinics of North America (ISSN 0889-8529) is published quarterly by Elsevier Inc., 360 Park Avenue South, New York, NY 10010-1710. Months of issue are March, June, September, and December. Periodicals postage paid at New York, NY and additional mailing offices. Subscription prices are USD 330.00 per year for US individuals, USD 581.00 per year for US institutions, USD 165.00 per year for US students and residents, USD 415.00 per year for Canadian individuals, USD 718.00 per year for Canadian institutions, USD 480.00 per year for international individuals, USD 718.00 per year for international institutions, and USD 245.00 per year for international and Canadian and foreign students/residents. To receive student/resident rate, orders must be accompanied by name of affiliated institution, date of term, and the signature of program/residency coordinator on institution letterhead. Orders will be billed at individual rate until proof of status is received. Foreign air speed delivery is included in all *Clinics* subscription prices. All prices are subject to change without notice. **POSTMASTER:** Send address changes to *Endocrinology and Metabolism Clinics of North America*, Elsevier Health Sciences Division, Subscription Customer Service, 3251 Riverport Lane, Maryland Heights, MO 63043. **Customer Service: Telephone: 1-800-654-2452** (U.S. and Canada); **1-314-447-8871** (outside U.S. and Canada). **Fax: 1-314-447-8029. E-mail: journalscustomerservice-usa@elsevier.com** (for print support); **journalsonlinesupport-usa@elsevier.com** (for online support).

Reprints. For copies of 100 or more, of articles in this publication, please contact the Commercial Rights Department, Elsevier Inc., 360 Park Avenue South, New York, NY 10010-1710; phone: +1-212-633-3874; fax: +1-212-633-3820; E-mail: reprints@elsevier.com.

Endocrinology and Metabolism Clinics of North America is covered in *MEDLINE/PubMed (Index Medicus), EMBASE/Excerpta Medica, Current Contents/Clinical Medicine, Current Contents/Life Sciences, Science Citation Index, ISI/BIOMED, BIOSIS*, and *Chemical Abstracts*.

Contributors

CONSULTING EDITOR

DEREK LEROITH, MD, PhD
Director of Research, Division of Endocrinology, Metabolism, and Bone Diseases, Department of Medicine, Mount Sinai School of Medicine, New York, New York

EDITORS

ANAT BEN-SHLOMO, MD
Associate Professor of Medicine, Pituitary Center, Division of Endocrinology, Diabetes and Metabolism, Department of Medicine, Cedars Sinai Medical Center, Los Angeles, California

MARIA FLESERIU, MD, FACE
Associate Professor; Director, Northwest Pituitary Center, Division of Endocrinology, Diabetes, and Clinical Nutrition, Departments of Medicine and Neurological Surgery, Oregon Health & Science University, Portland, Oregon

AUTHORS

PAULA BRUNA ARAUJO, MD
Endocrinology Section, Neuroendocrinology Research Center, Medical School and Hospital Universitário Clementino Fraga Filho, Universidade Federal do Rio de Janeiro, Rio de Janeiro, Rio de Janeiro, Brazil

RENATA S. AURIEMMA, MD
Ios-Coleman Medicina Futura Medical Center, Naples, Italy

ALBERT BECKERS, MD, PhD
Chief, Department of Endocrinology, Centre Hospitalier Universitaire de Liège, University of Liège, Liège, Belgium

ANAT BEN-SHLOMO, MD
Associate Professor of Medicine, Pituitary Center, Division of Endocrinology, Diabetes and Metabolism, Department of Medicine, Cedars Sinai Medical Center, Los Angeles, California

IGNACIO BERNABEU, MD
Endocrinology Division, Departamento de Medicina, Complejo Hospitalario Universitario de Santiago de Compostela, SERGAS, Universidad de Santiago de Compostela, Santiago de Compostela, Spain

MARTIN BIDLINGMAIER, MD
Head, Endocrine Research Unit, Medizinische Klinik und Poliklinik IV, Klinikum der Ludwig-Maximilians-Universität (LMU), Munich, Germany

CLAIRE BRIET, MD, PhD
Assistance Publique-Hôpitaux de Paris, Hôpital de Bicêtre, Department of Endocrinology and Reproductive Diseases, Le Kremlin-Bicêtre, France; University Paris-Sud, School of Medicine, Orsay, France

MARCELLO D. BRONSTEIN, MD, PhD
Neuroendocrine Unit, Laboratory of Cellular and Molecular Endocrinology LIM-25, Division of Endocrinology and Metabolism, Hospital das Clinicas, University of São Paulo Medical School, São Paulo, Brazil

CRISTINA CAPATINA, MD
Assistant Professor, Department of Endocrinology, C.I. Parhon National Institute of Endocrinology, Carol Davila University of Medicine and Pharmacy; Consultant, Department of Pituitary and Neuroendocrine Diseases, C.I. Parhon National Institute of Endocrinology, Bucharest, Romania

FELIPE F. CASANUEVA, MD, PhD
Endocrinology Division, Departamento de Medicina, Complejo Hospitalario Universitario de Santiago de Compostela, SERGAS, Universidad de Santiago de Compostela; Research Centre in Physiopathology of Obesity and Nutrition, Instituto Salud Carlos III, Santiago de Compostela, Spain

ANA I. CASTRO
Endocrinology Division, Departamento de Medicina, Complejo Hospitalario Universitario de Santiago de Compostela, SERGAS, Universidad de Santiago de Compostela; Research Centre in Physiopathology of Obesity and Nutrition, Instituto Salud Carlos III, Santiago de Compostela, Spain

PHILIPPE CHANSON, MD
Assistance Publique-Hôpitaux de Paris, Hôpital de Bicêtre, Department of Endocrinology and Reproductive Diseases, Le Kremlin-Bicêtre, France; University Paris-Sud, School of Medicine, Orsay, France; Institut National de la santé et de la Recherche Médicale, U693, Le Kremlin-Bicêtre, France

SILVIA CHIAVISTELLI, MD
Endocrinology, University of Brescia, Brescia, Italy

ANNAMARIA COLAO, MD, PhD
Professore, Dipartimento di Medicina Clinica e Chirurgia, Sezione di Endocrinologia, University "Federico II", Naples, Italy

IRIS CRESPO, MPsy
Departments of Endocrinology and Medicine, Hospital Sant Pau, Centro de Investigación Biomédica en Red de Enfermedades Raras (CIBER-ER, Unidad 747), IIB-Sant Pau, ISCIII, Universitat Autònoma de Barcelona (UAB), Barcelona, Spain

MICHAEL D. CUSIMANO, MD, PhD
Department of Neurosurgery, St. Michael's Hospital, University of Toronto, Toronto, Ontario, Canada

ROBERT F. DALLAPIAZZA, MD, PhD
Department of Neurosurgery, University of Virginia, Charlottesville, Virginia

ADRIAN F. DALY, MB BCh, PhD
Department of Endocrinology, Centre Hospitalier Universitaire de Liège, University of Liège, Liège, Belgium

ANTONIO DI IEVA, MD, PhD
Department of Neurosurgery, St. Michael's Hospital, University of Toronto, Toronto, Ontario, Canada

EVA FERNANDEZ-RODRIGUEZ, MD
Endocrinology Division, Departamento de Medicina, Complejo Hospitalario Universitario de Santiago de Compostela, SERGAS, Universidad de Santiago de Compostela, Santiago de Compostela, Spain

LUCIA FERRERI, MD
Dipartimento di Medicina Clinica e Chirurgia, Sezione di Endocrinologia, University "Federico II", Naples, Italy

MARIA FLESERIU, MD, FACE
Associate Professor; Director, Northwest Pituitary Center, Division of Endocrinology, Diabetes, and Clinical Nutrition, Departments of Medicine and Neurological Surgery, Oregon Health & Science University, Portland, Oregon

HIDENORI FUKUOKA, MD, PhD
Division of Diabetes and Endocrinology, Kobe University Hospital, Kobe, Japan

MÔNICA R. GADELHA, MD, PhD
Endocrinology Section, Neuroendocrinology Research Center, Medical School and Hospital Universitário Clementino Fraga Filho, Universidade Federal do Rio de Janeiro; Neuroendocrinology Unit, Instituto Estadual do Cérebro – Rua do Rezende, Rio de Janeiro, Brazil

ANDREA GIUSTINA, MD
Chair of Endocrinology, University of Brescia, Brescia, Italy

ANDREA GLEZER, MD, PhD
Neuroendocrine Unit, Laboratory of Cellular and Molecular Endocrinology LIM-25, Division of Endocrinology and Metabolism, Hospital das Clinicas, University of São Paulo Medical School, São Paulo, Brazil

JOHN A. JANE Jr, MD
Associate Professor, Department of Neurosurgery, University of Virginia, Charlottesville, Virginia

EMMANUEL JOUANNEAU, MD, PhD
INSERM U1028, CNRS UMR5292, Lyon Neuroscience Research Center, Neuro-Oncology & Neuro-Inflammation Team; University of Lyon 1, Lyon, France; Department of Neurosurgery, Groupement Hospitalier Est, Bron, France

RIIA K. JUNNILA, PhD
Postdoctoral Fellow, Endocrine Research Unit, Medizinische Klinik und Poliklinik IV, Klinikum der Ludwig-Maximilians-Universität (LMU), Munich, Germany

NIKI KARAVITAKI, MSc, PhD, FRCP
Department of Endocrinology, Oxford Centre for Diabetes, Endocrinology and Metabolism, Churchill Hospital, Headington, Oxford, United Kingdom

KALMAN KOVACS, MD, PhD
Division of Pathology, Department of Laboratory Medicine, St. Michael's Hospital, University of Toronto, Toronto, Ontario, Canada

SARAH E. MAYSON, MD
Assistant Professor of Medicine (Clinical), Division of Endocrinology, The Warren Alpert Medical School, Brown University, East Providence, Rhode Island

GHERARDO MAZZIOTTI, MD, PhD
Endocrinology, University of Brescia, Brescia, Italy

SHLOMO MELMED, MD
Pituitary Center, Cedars-Sinai Medical Center, Los Angeles, California

LEONARDO VIEIRA NETO, MD, PhD
Endocrinology Section, Neuroendocrinology Research Center, Medical School and Hospital Universitário Clementino Fraga Filho, Universidade Federal do Rio de Janeiro; Department of Endocrinology, Hospital Federal da Lagoa – Rua Jardim Botânico, Rio de Janeiro, Rio de Janeiro, Brazil

GEORGIA NTALI, MD, PhD
Department of Endocrinology, Oxford Centre for Diabetes, Endocrinology and Metabolism, Churchill Hospital, Headington, Oxford, United Kingdom

ROSARIO PIVONELLO, MD, PhD
Professore, Dipartimento di Medicina Clinica e Chirurgia, Sezione di Endocrinologia, University "Federico II", Naples, Italy

PRISCO PRISCITELLI, MD, PhD
Ios-Coleman Medicina Futura Medical Center, Naples, Italy

HERSHEL RAFF, PhD
Professor, Departments of Medicine, Surgery, and Physiology, Medical College of Wisconsin; Scientific Director and Clinical Supervisor, Endocrine Research Laboratory, Aurora St. Luke's Medical Center, Aurora Research Institute, Milwaukee, Wisconsin

GÉRALD RAVEROT, MD, PhD
INSERM U1028, CNRS UMR5292, Lyon Neuroscience Research Center, Neuro-Oncology & Neuro-Inflammation Team; University of Lyon 1, Lyon, France; Department of Endocrinology, Groupement Hospitalier Est, Hospices Civils de Lyon, Bron, France

FABIO ROTONDO, BSc
Division of Pathology, Department of Laboratory Medicine, St. Michael's Hospital, University of Toronto, Toronto, Ontario, Canada

SYLVIE SALENAVE, MD
Assistance Publique-Hôpitaux de Paris, Hôpital de Bicêtre, Department of Endocrinology and Reproductive Dieases, Le Kremlin-Bicêtre, France

ALICIA SANTOS, MPsy
Departments of Endocrinology and Medicine, Hospital Sant Pau, Centro de Investigación Biomédica en Red de Enfermedades Raras (CIBER-ER, Unidad 747), IIB-Sant Pau, ISCIII, Universitat Autònoma de Barcelona (UAB), Barcelona, Spain

AYDIN SAV, MD
Professor, Department of Pathology, Acibadem University, School of Medicine, Atasehir, Istanbul, Turkey

PETER J. SNYDER, MD
Professor of Medicine, Division of Endocrinology, Diabetes and Metabolism, Perelman School of Medicine, University of Pennsylvania, Philadelphia, Pennsylvania

CHRISTIAN J. STRASBURGER, MD
Professor of Medicine; Head of Clinical Endocrinology, Department of Endocrinology and Metabolic Diseases, Campus Charité Mitte, Charité Universitaetsmedizin, Berlin, Germany

LUIS V. SYRO, MD
Department of Neurosurgery, Hospital Pablo Tobon Uribe and Clinica Medellin, Medellin, Colombia

JACQUELINE TROUILLAS, MD, PhD
INSERM U1028, CNRS UMR5292, Lyon Neuroscience Research Center, Neuro-Oncology & Neuro-Inflammation Team; University of Lyon 1, Lyon, France; Department of Pathology, Groupement Hospitalier Est, Bron, France

ELENA VALASSI, MD, PhD
Departments of Endocrinology and Medicine, Hospital Sant Pau, Centro de Investigación Biomédica en Red de Enfermedades Raras (CIBER-ER, Unidad 747), IIB-Sant Pau, ISCIII, Universitat Autònoma de Barcelona (UAB), Barcelona, Spain

ALEXANDRE VASILJEVIC, MD
INSERM U1028, CNRS UMR5292, Lyon Neuroscience Research Center, Neuro-Oncology & Neuro-Inflammation Team; University of Lyon 1, Lyon, France; Department of Pathology, Groupement Hospitalier Est, Bron, France

JOHN A.H. WASS, MD, FRCP
Professor, Discipline of Endocrinology and Diabetes, University of Oxford; Senior Consultant, Department of Endocrinology, Oxford Centre for Diabetes, Endocrinology and Metabolism, Churchill Hospital, Headington, Oxford, United Kingdom

SUSAN M. WEBB, MD, PhD
Departments of Endocrinology and Medicine, Hospital Sant Pau, Centro de Investigación Biomédica en Red de Enfermedades Raras (CIBER-ER, Unidad 747), IIB-Sant Pau, ISCIII, Universitat Autònoma de Barcelona (UAB), Barcelona, Spain

Contents

> Pituitary tumors are commonly encountered intracranial neoplasms that are invariably benign. Classic oncogene mutations are not encountered in these tumors, and disrupted cell cycle control and growth factor signaling likely contribute to pathogenesis and natural history. They have unique clinical features that are determined by the secreted hormone gene product.

> Pituitary endocrine tumors are considered as benign. However, clinical and pathological data favor their consideration as more than an endocrinological disease. Using data from a retrospective case-control study of 410 patients, with 8 years of follow-up, the authors have validated a new clinicopathologic classification of pituitary tumors. This classification is based on tumor size, immunohistochemical type, and grade based on the assessment of invasion and proliferation, and it provides a prognostic value for predicting postoperative disease-free outcome or recurrence/progression status. This classification aids the identification of patients presenting with pituitary tumors that have a high risk of recurrence and enable construction of personalized therapies.

> The most frequent conditions that are associated with inherited/familial pituitary adenomas are familial isolated pituitary adenoma (FIPA) and multiple endocrine neoplasia type 1 (MEN1), which together account for up to 5% of pituitary adenomas. One important genetic cause of FIPA are inactivating mutations or deletions in the aryl hydrocarbon receptor interacting protein (*AIP*) gene. FIPA is the most frequent clinical presentation of *AIP* mutations. This article traces the current state of knowledge regarding the clinical features of FIPA and the particular genetic, pathologic, and clinical characteristics of pituitary adenomas due to *AIP* mutations.

Identifying the correct cause of hyperprolactinemia is crucial for treatment. Prolactinoma is the most common pathologic cause of hyperprolactinemia. Dopamine agonists are efficacious in about 80% to 90% of patients with prolactinoma, leading to reduction of serum prolactin levels and tumor dimensions. Neurosurgery, mainly by the transsphenoidal route, is indicated in cases of intolerant and resistant dopamine agonists. Radiotherapy is rarely used because of its side effects and low efficacy. The alkylating agent temozolomide showed efficacy for treatment of aggressive and resistant prolactinomas. Other approaches, such as thyrosine kinase inhibitors, are currently being tested and could be an additional tool for these troublesome tumors.

Pituitary adenomas are frequently silent. Among silent adenomas, some are clinically silent but can be detected on the basis of the excessive secretion of hormonal products, whereas others are totally silent and cannot be detected by hormonal measurements. Treatment of a silent pituitary adenoma depends on its size and extent. Silent adenomas that are associated with neurologic compromise should be treated by surgery. Postoperative radiation therapy may be used to prevent or treat recurrences. Only occasional silent pituitary adenomas respond to treatment with dopamine agonists or somatostatin analogs.

Cabergoline (CAB) is widely used for the medical treatment of pituitary tumors, particularly those associated with hormone hypersecretion. Whether treatment with CAB is associated with an increased risk of clinically relevant cardiac valve disease in patients with pituitary tumors is still debated. In most studies, CAB has been found not associated with an increased risk of significant valvulopathy, and no correlation has been shown between valvular abnormalities and CAB duration or cumulative dose. This review provides an overview of the studies reporting on the outcome of CAB in terms of cardiac valve disease in patients with pituitary tumors.

Aggressive pituitary adenomas have a high risk of recurrence, a lack of therapeutic response, and resistance to conventional treatment. So far, no satisfactory biomarkers are available for predicting their behavior. Some specific pituitary adenoma histotypes are more prone to follow an aggressive behavior. Pituitary carcinomas are rare and show cerebrospinal and/or systemic metastasis. They have worse prognosis than aggressive adenomas, and radiation is of limited use in their treatment.

of anterior hypopituitarism of 27.5%. Growth hormone deficiency is the most prevalent hormone insufficiency after TBI; however, the prevalence of each type of pituitary deficiency is influenced by the assays used for diagnosis, severity of head trauma, and time of evaluation. Recent studies have demonstrated improvement in cognitive function and cognitive quality of life with substitution therapy in GH-deficient patients after TBI.

In the last 15 years, worse health-related quality of life (QoL) has been reported in patients with pituitary diseases compared with healthy individuals. Different QoL questionnaires have shown incomplete physical and psychological recovery after therapy. Residual impairments often affect QoL even long-term after successful treatment of pituitary adenomas. In this article, knowledge of factors that affect QoL in pituitary diseases is reviewed. The focus is on 5 pituitary diseases: Cushing syndrome, acromegaly, prolactinomas, nonfunctioning pituitary adenomas, and hypopituitarism.

Pituitary hormones have direct and indirect effects on bone remodeling, and skeletal fragility is a frequent complication of pituitary diseases. Fragility fractures may occur in many patients with prolactinomas, acromegaly, Cushing disease, and hypopituitarism. As in other forms of secondary osteoporosis, pituitary diseases generally affect bone quality more than bone quantity, and fractures may occur even in the presence of normal or low-normal bone mineral density, making difficult the prediction of fractures in these settings. Treatment of excess and defective pituitary hormone generally improves skeletal health, although some patients remain at high risk for fractures, necessitating treatment with bone-active drugs.

The improved management of pituitary adenomas has led to an increasing number of pregnancies in patients harboring pituitary adenomas. Therefore, adequate management of pregnant women with pituitary adenomas is of growing importance. Because pregnancy produces several physiologic changes to the endocrine system, especially to the pituitary gland, endocrinologists must be knowledgeable and skilled to effectively manage pregnant women with pituitary adenomas and to guarantee the wellbeing of the fetus.

Pituitary apoplexy (PA) is a rare clinical syndrome caused by sudden hemorrhaging and/or infarction of the pituitary gland, generally within a pituitary adenoma. The main symptom is sudden-onset severe headache, associated with visual disorders or ocular palsy. Corticotropic deficiency may be

ENDOCRINOLOGY AND METABOLISM CLINICS OF NORTH AMERICA

Foreword

Pituitary Disorders

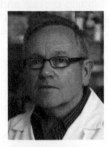

Derek LeRoith, MD, PhD
Consulting Editor

This issue on Pituitary Disorders comprises a larger number of articles than usual and is an indication of new and interesting discoveries in the field. The articles, as is standard in this series, describe both basic aspects of the disorders and practical, clinical approaches to dealing with these disorders.

In the opening article of this issue, Dr Shlomo Melmed presents an overview of the topic of pituitary tumors, describing the six types of tumors according to the cell of origin and the syndrome of hormone excess associated with each one. The hormones include ACTH, GH, TSH, prolactin, and gonadotrophins (FSH and LH); the last two are not associated with hormonal excess syndrome. Generally, the tumors are benign, and the article covers the many signaling and transcription factors involved in the progression of the tumors and the secretion of the hormones as well as some of the signs and symptoms associated with each tumor.

Drs Raverot, Vasiljevic, Jouanneau, and Trouillas describe a new concept in the classification of pituitary tumors based on both clinical and pathologic findings. They posit, from over 400 patients with pituitary tumors, that certain pathologic findings are predictive of postoperative disease-free outcomes and, most importantly, the recurrence of the disorder. The features that determine these results include the pathologic staging of the tumor, including invasiveness, as well as men with GH-, ACTH-, or prolactin-producing tumors. Thus, with further studies like these, we may be able to enter into the realm of "personalized medicine."

An unusual subtype of pituitary adenomas is caused by germline mutations or deletions in the aryl hydrocarbon receptor interacting protein gene. This results in "familial isolated pituitary tumors," that present as either the same subtype of tumor (homozygous gene defect) or different subtypes in the same family (heterozygous gene defect). As discussed by Drs Daly and Beckers, these tumors may present in younger individuals in the family and are often GH-secreting tumors that are relatively resistant to somatostatin analogue therapy.

Endocrinol Metab Clin N Am 44 (2015) xvii–xx
http://dx.doi.org/10.1016/j.ecl.2014.12.002
0889-8529/15/$ – see front matter © 2015 Published by Elsevier Inc.

endo.theclinics.com

The accurate diagnosis of excess or impaired growth is dependent on the measurement of circulating GH and IGF-1 levels. Furthermore, response to therapy and adjustment of therapeutic agents often rely on these measurements. Drs Junnila, Strasburger, and Bidlingmaier discuss the pitfalls inherent in the laboratory measurements. Factors affecting GH assays include the presence of GH-binding protein and reduced GH levels in obesity. For GH deficiency, the most accurate testing is GHRH/arginine combined stimulation, and for excess GH, the use of an oral glucose tolerance test. Standardization of GH assays can be achieved between laboratories by the use of the same antibodies and similar units to express the results. Similarly, with the IGF-1 assay, IGFBPs must be dealt with appropriately. Recently "free" IGF-1 assays have been developed, although their accuracy and value are still in question; indeed, total IGF-1 remains the gold standard and tracks GH biological action very closely.

Surgery is generally recommended for the treatment of acromegaly. Where surgery is not possible or more commonly has failed to completely reverse the excess GH secretion, medical therapy is indicated. To date, the medical therapies include somatostatin receptor ligands (octreotide and lanreotide), pegvisomant, and dopamine agonists. More recently, Dr Ben-Shlomo describes a new a new somatostatin receptor ligand with binding affinity to SST5>SST2>SST3>SST1, pasireotide, that has been tested in clinical trials. Although it has shown promise as an alternative, the concern is the increased incidence of hyperglycemia and frank diabetes in a greater percentage of individuals on this new agent.

Dr Raff discusses the difficulties that endocrinologists encounter with the diagnosis of Cushing disease. Until recently, standard tests, such as serum-free cortisol or 24-hour urinary cortisol, each had their own problems for screening individuals who presented with features compatible with the condition. Overnight low-dose dexamethasone suppression tests became the standard until, over the past decade, late-night salivary cortisol replaced it as the "gold standard" for screening, because of its high degree of sensitivity and specificity. Another update described in this article is the use of prolactin measurements when performing inferior petrosal sinus sampling to ensure the correct placement of the catheters. This becomes important when using the technique to distinguish extopic ACTH from pituitary Cushing.

Cushing disease is usually treated with transphenoidal surgery. When inadequately "cured," medical therapy is appropriate. A number of options are available, including pasireotide, that inhibits ACTH secretion, although it often causes hyperglycemia and frank diabetes. Because corticotroph adenomas simultaneously express Sstr5 and dopamine D2 receptors, pasireotide could be combined with cabergoline, a dopamine antagonist. Mifepristone can be used in patients with diabetes but should be avoided in those with more severe hypertension and accompanying hypokalemia. Adrenal steroidogenesis inhibitors (ketoconazole and metyrapone), although not approved, have proven valuable in some patients. As discussed by Dr Fleseriu, combination therapy may allow for improved responses and may avoid the option of adrenalectomy in the more resistant patients with Cushing disease.

Drs Glezer and Bronstein, in their article, discuss prolactinomas and remind us that hyperprolactinemia is one of the most common causes of infertility in both men and women. Although prolactinoma is a common cause, hyperprolactinemia can be caused by multiple other medical conditions and drugs. Typically, treatment with dopamine agonists is successful in controlling the prolactin levels and even reducing the tumor size; however, transphenoidal removal may be indicated.

Silent or nonfunctional pituitary adenomas may arise from any cell type, although more commonly they are gonadotropin in origin. To confirm that they are nonfunctional requires a full hormonal evaluation. As discussed by Drs Mayson and Snyder, these adenomas are either found incidentally or present with neurologic symptoms due to pressure effects. In the latter case, they require surgical removal with very occasional radiotherapy. Follow-up hormonal evaluation is critical because hypopituitarism may follow surgical removal of the adenoma because of damage to adjacent normal pituitary tissue. There are some tumors that may respond to dopamine agonists or somatostatin analogues, although often not to a clinically significant degree.

Drs Auriemma, Pivonello, Ferreri, Priscitelli, and Colao discuss the concern that arose with the use of cabergoline for the management of prolactinomas as well as acromegaly. Cabergoline use in Parkinson disorder was associated with cardiac valvular changes requiring interventional therapy. However, as these authors describe in this article, there is no evidence that similar side effects have been detected with its use at regular dosing in treating prolactinomas. However, when used at much higher doses, caution is warranted, and cardiac screening using echocardiography is always appropriate under these circumstances. In the case of nonfunctioning tumors and Cushing patients, no studies have been described.

Pituitary adenomas are generally nonaggressive; however, some may show manifestations of more aggressive behavior. Unfortunately, no biomarkers can distinguish between these two situations, and pathologic changes are often helpful. As Drs Sav, Rotondo, Syro, Di Ieva, Cusimano, and Kovacs discuss, the aggressive tumors often manifest with clinically relevant features, such as a high risk of recurrence and resistance to therapy. In addition, they describe the rare occurrence of pituitary carcinomas, with spread to the cerebrospinal fluid space, and even systemic metastasis.

Removal of pituitary tumors, both functioning and nonfunctioning, is performed by traditional microscopic transsphenoidal surgery. Drs Dallapiazza and Jane describe the introduction of endoscopic transsphenoidal surgery that enables the surgeon to have a more panoramic view of the larger tumors with more lighting. However, in the hands of experienced surgeons, both techniques are equally effective.

Radiation therapy is usually used for sellar and parasellar tumors, especially when surgery has been less than totally successful. As outlined in the article by Drs Ntali and Karavitaki, the main long-term complications include hypopituitarism, optic neuropathy, cerebrovascular morbidity, and second brain tumors. These side effects of radiation are often determined by the type and intensity of the radiation used.

Drs Wass and Capatina describe the central loss of GH and ACTH deficiency. Often, these deficiencies are the result of tumors in the region of the hypothalamic and pituitary regions. GH deficiency is associated with increased cardiovascular risk; alterations in substrate metabolism; and impaired body composition, muscle strength, bone mass, and quality of life (QOL). It requires dynamic testing for the diagnosis and can be treated by replacing GH. It is not immediately life-threatening in contrast to ACTH deficiency, otherwise known as central adrenal insufficiency. In this case, glucocorticoid replacement is critical and lifelong and often requires increased dosing during severe stress situations.

Hypophysitis may be primary or secondary, the former due to IgG_4-related and the latter due to anticytotoxic T-lymphocyte antigen-4 antibodies. Clinically, one may see sellar mass effects, hypopituitarism, central diabetes insipidus, or hyperprolactinemia. Dr Fukuoka describes the clinical-pathologic features, the diagnosis, and management of the condition; management often requires reduction of the sellar mass and hormonal replacement therapy.

Hypopituitarism commonly follows traumatic brain injury, often more commonly than previously appreciated. Drs Fernandez-Rodriguez, Bernabeu, Castro, and

Casanueva explain that ACTH loss is often the only hormonal deficiency that, if detected early, fails to recover, whereas the others may recover. GH is the most common deficiency after TBI, and GH replacement may improve cognitive dysfunction seen in these cases.

Drs Crespo, Valassi, Santos, and Webb remind us that QOL is severely affected in pituitary tumors with excess hormone secretion as well as after therapy of the tumors. Hypopituitarism is similarly a major factor in this poor QOL in our patients, and we, as physicians, need to pay more attention to this problem even as we work to achieve normal hormonal homeostasis.

It is well established that disorders of both excess and deficiency of pituitary hormones affect bone quality and lead to an increase in bone fractures. Drs Mazziotti, Chiavistelli, and Giustina explain that these fractures are often fragile in nature and therefore not readily detected by standard dual-energy X-ray absorptiometry. Fortunately, replacement of deficient hormones or reduction in the excess hormone syndromes often restores bone quality. However, because this restoration may not be complete, often the physician has to resort to using bone-active drugs to prevent the increased risk of fractures.

The management of pituitary tumors in pregnancy is understandably complex. Microadenomas seldom enlarge during pregnancy, whereas macroadenomas are prone to do so. When indicated, surgical removal should be performed in the second trimester. Generally, if patients are on therapies for their tumors, the therapy is stopped upon the establishment of the pregnancy, unless the tumor is encroaching the optic chiasm; an individualized decision will then have to made. Drs Araujo, Viero Neto, and Dadelha discuss how Cushing disease is extremely challenging because the excess cortisol leads to a high-risk pregnancy.

In the final article, Drs Chanson, Briet, and Salenave discuss pituitary apoplexy, a fairly uncommon occurrence where hemorrhaging occurs in a pituitary adenoma. Clinically, it often presents with the sudden onset of a severe headache, associated with visual disorders or ocular palsy. The marked decrease in glucocorticoid levels may be life-threatening, and early treatment with glucocorticoids is essential. Although neurosurgical intervention may be warranted in some cases, conservative therapy is often chosen. In the long term, many if not most pituitary hormones are found to be reduced and require replacement.

I sincerely hope that the readers enjoy this issue as much as I did and appreciate the contributions by experts in the field. Special thanks are due to our issue editors, Drs Ben-Shlomo and Fleseriu, for an outstanding job.

Derek LeRoith, MD, PhD
Director of Research
Division of Endocrinology, Metabolism, and Bone Diseases
Department of Medicine
Mount Sinai School of Medicine
One Gustave L. Levy Place
Box 1055, Altran 4-36
New York, NY 10024, USA

E-mail address:
derek.leroith@mssm.edu

Preface

Updates and Highlights in Pituitary Medicine

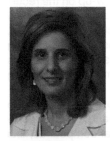 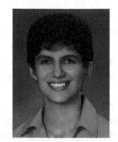

Anat Ben-Shlomo, MD   Maria Fleseriu, MD, FACE
Editors

Pituitary diseases are relatively rare and often manifest with pleomorphic and vague clinical features commonly overlapping with those of other, more common diseases. As a result, pituitary diseases are often overlooked by health care providers, leading to missed or late diagnosis and increased burden of illness on patients, physicians, and the health care system. Moreover, misinterpretation of disease status and inappropriate treatment are frequent and can lead to increased morbidity and mortality in this unique subgroup of patients.

When filtered by the terms "pituitary gland," "pituitary adenoma," or "pituitary tumor," more than 5000 publications have been documented in PubMed since 2008, the year in which the last special issue of Pituitary Disorders (edited by Dr Ariel Barkan) was published in *Endocrinology and Metabolism Clinics of North America*, quite a plethora for such a rare set of diseases. Indeed, significant progress in our understanding of pituitary tumor pathophysiology, diagnosis, and treatment has occurred over the last 6 years.

Several important pathways in the pathogenesis of pituitary tumors have been unraveled. The role of cyclin E and EGFR signaling in pituitary adenoma formation and progression was elucidated, leading to new clinical trials with relevant inhibitors. Multiple germline mutations or deletions in the aryl hydrocarbon receptor interacting protein gene were shown to be involved in the pathogenesis of familial isolated pituitary adenomas and pituitary adenoma, gigantism, and apoplexy in young patients. Novel IgG$_4$-related hypophysitis and secondary hypophysitis due to treatment with anticytotoxic T-lymphocyte antigen-4 antibodies have been described. Traumatic brain injury and pituitary apoplexy have been increasingly recognized as important causes of hypopituitarism.

Endocrinol Metab Clin N Am 44 (2015) xxi–xxiii
http://dx.doi.org/10.1016/j.ecl.2014.12.001
0889-8529/15/$ – see front matter © 2015 Published by Elsevier Inc.

endo.theclinics.com

Pituitary Tumors

Shlomo Melmed, MD

KEYWORDS

- Pituitary • Tumor • Neoplasm • Hormone gene products

KEY POINTS

- Pituitary tumors are commonly encountered intracranial neoplasms that are invariably benign.
- Classic oncogene mutations are not encountered in these tumors, and disrupted cell cycle control and growth factor signaling likely contribute to pathogenesis and natural history.
- Pituitary tumors have unique clinical features that are determined by the secreted hormone gene product.

Anterior pituitary cell types express distinct hormone gene products. These products include adrenocorticotropic hormone (ACTH), growth hormone (GH), prolactin (PRL), thyroid-stimulating hormone (TSH), follicle-stimulating hormone (FSH), and luteinizing hormone (LH). Pituitary adenomas are distinguished by excess proliferation of one of these differentiated cell types, as well as dysregulated specific hormone hypersecretion. Physiologically, the 6 pituitary trophic hormones regulate respective target hormone production and endocrine gland function in tightly controlled regulatory loops (**Fig. 1**). Adenoma hypersecretion is usually a reflection of dysregulated hormone synthesis and/or secretion.

Each of these cell-specific adenomas is associated with a benign sellar mass, as well as a unique clinical syndrome associated with the hormone being hypersecreted.[1] Thus, lactotroph adenomas result in hyperprolactinemia, with features of hypogonadism accompanied by galactorrhea. Corticotroph adenomas hypersecrete ACTH, leading to features of hypercortisolism associated with central obesity, hypertension, hyperglycemia, infections, and psychological disturbances. Somatotroph adenomas hypersecrete GH, leading to features of acromegaly, including acral changes, arthritis, hypertension, headache, soft tissue swelling, and hyperglycemia. Thyrotroph adenomas hypersecreting TSH are extremely rare, and may be associated with mild hyperthyroidisms and goiter. Tumors arising from gonadotroph cells rarely hypersecrete intact FSH or LH, and more commonly express either glycoprotein subunits or no excess hormone. These adenomas are often discovered incidentally, and are

Disclosures: Dr S. Melmed has received research funding from the NIH.
Pituitary Center, Cedars-Sinai Medical Center, 8700 Beverly Boulevard, Room 2015, Los Angeles, CA 90048, USA
E-mail address: melmed@cshs.org

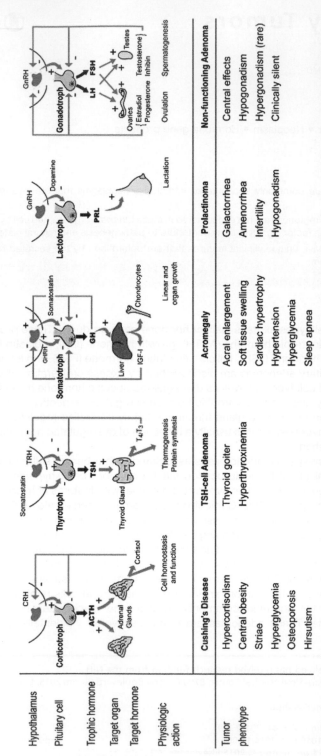

Fig. 1. Hormone secretion from pituitary tumors, although excessive and associated with unique phenotypic features, often retains intact trophic control. For example, dopaminergic agents appropriately suppress PRL secretion by prolactinomas, and dexamethasone may suppress ACTH secretion in patients with pituitary Cushing disease. (*From* Melmed S. Mechanisms for pituitary tumorigenesis: the plastic pituitary. J Clin Invest 2003;112: 1603–18; with permission.)

usually associated with hypogonadism and pituitary failure caused by compressive effects of the expanding mass (**Table 1**).

These adenomas, regardless of cell type, are invariably benign. Although often locally aggressive and invasive, they rarely progress to true malignancy with documented extracranial metastases.[2] Mechanisms underlying the constraints buffering pituitary adenomas against malignant transformation include development of DNA damage and premature proliferative arrest (ie, cell senescence). Senescent pituitary cells are growth constrained by cyclin-dependent kinase (CDK) inhibitors, including p21 for somatotroph tumors, p27 for corticotroph tumors, and p15/p165 for nonfunctioning adenomas.[3] These CDK inhibitors lead to cell cycle arrest while maintaining differentiated hormone secretion and preventing the malignant transformation of respective adenoma cell types.

Another pathogenetic feature of these tumors is their monoclonality.[4] Because pituitary tumors seem to arise from a single cell, it is unlikely that broad, generalized signals such as hypothalamic hormone excess, or estrogen excess, lead to polyclonal hyperplasia with resultant hormone hypersecretion. In support of this postulate, activating mutations of hypothalamic hormone receptors in pituitary adenomas (GH-releasing hormone receptor [GHRHR], corticotropin-C–releasing hormone receptor [CRHR], gonadotrophin-releasing hormone receptor [GnRHR], thyrotropin-releasing hormone receptor [TRHR]) have not been reported. Inactivating mutations of hypothalamic inhibitory factor receptors (SSTR1-5; D2R) similarly have not been reported. Consistent with these observations, adenoma monoclonality is also suggested by surgical resection of small (<10 mm), discrete, hormone-secreting adenomas (especially those expressing GH or ACTH) possibly resulting in long-term remission with sustained hormonal control. Note that pituitary tissue surrounding the adenoma does not show features of hyperplasia, further suggesting the discrete monocellular pathogenesis of these adenomas.

Multiple extracellular and intracellular signals determine pituitary cell proliferation and specific hormone synthesis and secretion (**Fig. 2**). Mitogenic hormones (eg, hypothalamic GH-releasing hormone [GHRH], corticotropin-C–releasing hormone [CRH], or gonadotrophin-releasing hormone) or growth factors (eg, epidermal growth factor) or steroids (eg estrogen) may induce pituitary cell proliferation as well as transcription of pituitary hormone genes. These mitogenic inputs are balanced by important constraining factors of pituitary cell proliferation and hormone synthesis, including hypothalamic somatostatin and dopamine. Hormones and growth factors also drive the cell cycle mediated by CDK-cyclin complexes and Rb phosphorylation. Release of E2F by phosphorylated Rb acts to drive cell cycle progression. This complex process is disrupted in adenomas, leading to chromosomal instability and DNA damage.[5] Pituitary adenomas are remarkably aneuploidy despite their benign phenotypes. Dysregulated hormone gene transcription occurs pari passu with cell proliferative changes.[6] It is apparent that disruption or activation of multiple sites within the hormone-secreting adenoma cell leads to the dual outcome of adenoma formation with subsequent proliferation, associated with a unique hormone hypersecretory phenotype.

ANIMAL MODELS

Although classic oncogene mutations are not encountered in sporadic tumors, several growth factor, hormone, and cell cycle genes are reported to determine development of sporadic pituitary adenomas.[7] Many have been tested in genetically modified mice, which either show gain of function or loss of function (**Table 2**). For example, heterozygote Rb$^{+/-}$ mutant mice develop pituitary adenomas with high penetrance, usually

Table 1
Classification of pituitary adenomas

Cell Type	Population Prevalence (Total/10^5)	Tumor Transcription Factor Expression	Upregulated Differentiated Gene Expression	Clinical Features
Lactotroph: sparsely or densely granulated	45–50	Pit-1	PRL	Hypogonadism and/or galactorrhea
Gonadotroph	15–20	SF-1, GATA-2	FSH and/or LH and/or glycoprotein subunit. (depending on type, null or oncocytic)	Silent or pituitary failure Ovarian hyperstimulation (reproductive-age women) Testicular enlargement (prepubertal)
Somatotroph	10	Pit-1	—	—
Sparsely granulated	—	—	GH	Acromegaly or gigantism
Densely granulated	—	—	GH	Acromegaly
Combined GH and PRL cells	—	—	GH and PRL	Acromegaly or gigantism
Mixed GH and PRL	—	—	GH and PRL	Hypogonadism and acromegaly
Mammosomatotroph	—	—	GH and PRL	Acromegaly or gigantism
Acidophil Stem Cell	—	—	PRL and GH	Hypogonadism and acromegaly
Silent	—	—	GH	Hypopituitarism
Corticotroph	5	T-Pit	ACTH	—
Cushing	—	—	—	Cushing disease
Silent	—	—	—	Hypopituitarism
Nelson	—	—	—	Pituitary hyperplasia
Thyrotroph	<1	Pit-1	TSH	Hyperthyroidism
Plurihormonal	Unknown	All	GH, PRL, ACTH, glycoprotein	Mixed

All tumor types show features of a pituitary mass, visible on MRI. Glycoprotein refers to intact FSH or LH, or respective alpha or beta glycoprotein subunits. Although null-cell tumors do not express hormone genes, they are classified as gonadotroph in origin.

Abbreviations: GATA2, endothelial transcription factor GATA-2; PIT1, pituitary-specific positive transcription factor 1; STF1, steroidogenic factor 1; TBX19, T-box transcription factor TBX19 (also known as TPIT).

From Melmed S. Pathogenesis of pituitary tumors. Nat Rev Endocrinol 2011;7:257–66; with permission.

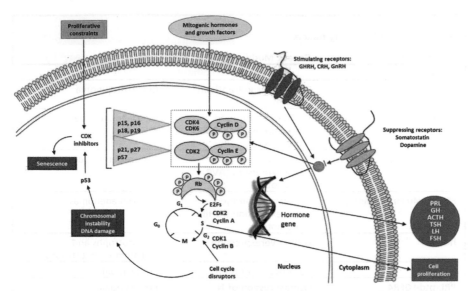

Fig. 2. Pituitary adenoma signaling. Transcription of pituitary hormone genes and cell proliferation are induced by pituitary mitogenic factors, including hypothalamic hormones and transcription factors, as well as peripheral hormones. Proliferative constraints include somatostatin and dopamine, as well as tumor suppressor genes. Cell cycle progression is mediated by CDK-cyclin complexes that phosphorylate Rb and cause it to release E2F, which drives cell proliferation. CDK inhibitors block kinase phosphorylation, thereby restraining cell cycle progression. Chromosomal instability, DNA damage, and senescence may act to constrain malignant transformation of pituitary tumors. (*From* Melmed S. Pathogenesis of pituitary tumors. Nat Rev Endocrinol 2011;7:257–66; with permission.)

arising from the intermediate lobe with overexpressed pro-opiomelanocortin (POMC).[8] Although several reported transgenic knock-in, universal knockout, and conditional knockout mice may faithfully recapitulate human phenotypes with specific cell type adenoma development and hormone hypersecretion, few such models have yielded a viable therapeutic drug discovery.

Transgenic overexpression or disruption of several cell cycle–associated genes have been observed to uniquely lead to pituitary tumor formation in several animal models (**Table 3**). These experimental tumors show varying degrees of penetrance, may be located in the anterior or intermediate lobes, and may or may not hypersecrete specific trophic hormones with resultant peripheral hormonal phenotypes. Two examples are presented of how further unraveling pituitary tumor signaling pathways in transgenic animal models may lead to translational discovery of novel subcellular therapeutic targets:

Targeting Cyclin-dependent Kinase Signaling

Pituitary tumor transforming gene (PTTG), isolated from rat pituitary tumor cells, is the index mammalian securin, and drives pituitary tumor formation in murine and zebra fish models.[9] The gene is also induced by estrogen in experimental prolactinomas[10] and is overexpressed in human pituitary tumor cells.[11] In an attempt to recreate an ACTH-secreting pituitary adenoma, the zebra fish *Pttg* gene was linked to the POMC promoter to create a corticotroph-targeted transgene. Transgenic zebra fish expressing pituitary corticotroph-directed *zpttg* develop phenotypic features that recapitulate human Cushing disease. These features include cortico-troph hyperplasia, hypercortisolism, hyperglycemia and fatty liver, and cardiac effu-sions and hypertrophy.[12] Furthermore, partial glucocorticoid resistance was also shown. Using this animal model as a drug therapy screening target, the transgenic zebra fish model was used for screening of small molecules showing specific CDK inhibitory activity in the hyperplastic transgenic pituitary. Accordingly, R-roscovi-tine, a selective CDK inhibitor, was shown to suppress tumorous pituitary POMC gene expression and ACTH secretion in both zebra fish and murine models of ACTH-secreting corticotroph cell adenomas. The drug also reversed phenotypic features in tumor-bearing mice. Suppressive effects of R-roscovitine on ACTH secretion were also recapitulated in cell cultures derived from resected human pi-tuitary tumor specimens.[12] Based on these translational studies elucidating mech-anisms for pituitary tumorigenesis, R-roscovitine has now been approved to enter clinical trials to test for safety and efficacy in patients with ACTH-secreting pituitary adenomas and Cushing disease.

Targeting Erb Signaling

Mechanisms underlying prolactinoma pathogenesis are challenging to elucidate because of the unavailability of functional PRL-secreting human pituitary tumor cell lines, as well as the shortage of available pituitary tumor tissue specimens. Both ErbB family receptors and ligands are expressed in normal anterior pituitary cells. Acti-vation of this signaling pathway leads to induced PRL production by regulating PRL gene expression and lactotroph differentiation.[13] To further elucidate mechanisms un-derlying prolactinoma tumorigenesis, transgenic mice expressing EGF receptor (EGFR) or human EGF receptor 2 (HER2) driven by the tissue-specific rPRL enhancer/promoter to achieve pituitary overexpression were generated. Lactotroph-targeted murine transgenic human EGFR (hEGFR)/HER2 expression induced murine prolactinomas secreting high PRL levels. When EGFR/HER2 activity was inhibited by treating mice with lapatinib, a dual tyrosine kinase inhibitor (TKI) for both EGFR and HER2, hyperprolactinemia and tumor mitogen-activated protein kinase (MAPK) and Akt pathways were attenuated.[14]

Furthermore, ACTH-secreting murine AtT20 cells and primary human cell cultures derived from resected ACTH-secreting tumors were suppressed by TKI treatment. In ATCH-secreting AtT20 cells, overexpression of EGFR led to activation of MAPK-Erk signaling, which was inhibited by gefitinib, an EGFR TKI.[15]

These observations provide a compelling rationale for the feasibility of using ErbB tar-geted therapy for patients with prolactinomas and those with Cushing disease. In a pilot clinical study, lapatinib was shown to attenuate PRL secretion in 2 patients harboring aggressive prolactinoma that was resistant to high-dose dopamine agonist therapy.[16]

SUMMARY

Pituitary tumors are commonly encountered intracranial neoplasms that are invariably benign. Classic oncogene mutations are not encountered in these tumors, and disrup-ted cell cycle control and growth factor signaling likely contribute to pathogenesis and natural history. They have unique clinical features that are determined by the secreted hormone gene product.

REFERENCES

1. Melmed S. Mechanisms for pituitary tumorigenesis: the plastic pituitary. J Clin Invest 2003;112:1603–18.

2. Chesnokova V, Zhou C, Ben-Shlomo A, et al. Growth hormone is a cellular senescence target in pituitary and nonpituitary cells. Proc Natl Acad Sci U S A 2013; 110:E3331–9.
3. Chesnokova V, Zonis S, Zhou C, et al. Lineage-specific restraint of pituitary gonadotroph cell adenoma growth. PLoS One 2011;6:e17924.
4. Herman V, Fagin J, Gonsky R, et al. Clonal origin of pituitary adenomas. J Clin Endocrinol Metab 1990;71:1427–33.
5. Chesnokova V, Zonis S, Kovacs K, et al. p21(Cip1) restrains pituitary tumor growth. Proc Natl Acad Sci U S A 2008;105:17498–503.
6. Melmed S. Acromegaly pathogenesis and treatment. J Clin Invest 2009;119: 3189–202.
7. Melmed S. Pathogenesis of pituitary tumors. Nat Rev Endocrinol 2011;7:257–66.
8. Jacks T. Tumor suppressor gene mutations in mice. Annu Rev Genet 1996;30: 603–36.
9. Pei L, Melmed S. Isolation and characterization of a pituitary tumor-transforming gene (PTTG). Mol Endocrinol 1997;11:433–41.
10. Heaney AP, Fernando M, Melmed S. Functional role of estrogen in pituitary tumor pathogenesis. J Clin Invest 2002;109:277–83.
11. Vlotides G, Eigler T, Melmed S. Pituitary tumor-transforming gene: physiology and implications for tumorigenesis. Endocr Rev 2007;28:165–86.
12. Liu NA, Jiang H, Ben-Shlomo A, et al. Targeting zebrafish and murine pituitary corticotroph tumors with a cyclin-dependent kinase (CDK) inhibitor. Proc Natl Acad Sci U S A 2011;108:8414–9.
13. Murdoch GH, Potter E, Nicolaisen AK, et al. Epidermal growth factor rapidly stimulates prolactin gene transcription. Nature 1982;300:192–4.
14. Liu X, Kano M, Araki T, et al. ErbB receptor-driven prolactinomas respond to targeted lapatinib treatment in female transgenic mice. Endocrinology 2014. [Epub ahead of print].
15. Fukuoka H, Cooper O, Ben-Shlomo A, et al. EGFR as a therapeutic target for human, canine, and mouse ACTH-secreting pituitary adenomas. J Clin Invest 2011;121:4712–21.
16. Cooper O, Mamelak A, Bannykh S, et al. Prolactinoma ErbB receptor expression and targeted therapy for aggressive tumors. Endocrine 2014;46:318–27.

A Prognostic Clinicopathologic Classification of Pituitary Endocrine Tumors

Gérald Raverot, MD, PhD[a,b,c], Alexandre Vasiljevic, MD[a,b,d],
Emmanuel Jouanneau, MD, PhD[a,b,e],
Jacqueline Trouillas, MD, PhD[a,b,d],*

KEYWORDS

- Classification • Pituitary endocrine tumor • Pathologic markers

KEY POINTS

- Clinicopathologic classification of endocrine pituitary tumors should take into account the immunohistochemical (IHC) type, the tumor size, and a grade based on the assessment of the invasion (by magnetic resonance imaging [MRI]) and the proliferation (evaluated by the mitotic count, the Ki-67, and p53 labeling).
- Some evidences suggest that the silent growth hormone (GH) or adrenocorticotropic hormone (ACTH) tumor and the prolactin (PRL) tumor in men are more often aggressive, but larger series are required.
- Somatostatin receptor (SSTR)$_2$ and SSTR$_5$ expression in GH and ACTH tumors could guide the therapeutic strategies.
- At present, systemic metastasis is needed to diagnose pituitary carcinoma, but recent data suggested that invasive and proliferative pituitary tumors should be considered as tumors suspected of malignancy.

This work was supported by grants from the Ministère de la Santé (Programme Hospitalier de Recherche Clinique National n°27-43 HYPOPRONOS and n°12-096 PITUIGENE) and research contracts with the National Institute of Health and Medical Research and the Ligue Contre le Cancer Rhône-Alpes.

[a] INSERM U1028, CNRS UMR5292, Lyon Neuroscience Research Center, Neuro-Oncology & Neuro-Inflammation Team, Lyon F-69372, France; [b] University of Lyon 1, Lyon F-69372, France; [c] Department of Endocrinology, Groupement Hospitalier Est, Hospices Civils de Lyon, 59 Boulevard Pinel, Bron F-69677, France; [d] Department of Pathology, Groupement Hospitalier Est, 59 Boulevard Pinel, Bron F-69677, France; [e] Department of Neurosurgery, Groupement Hospitalier Est, 59 Boulevard Pinel, Bron F-69677, France
* Corresponding author. INSERM U1028, CNRS UMR5292, Lyon Neuroscience Research Center, Neuro-Oncology & Neuro-Inflammation Team, University of Lyon 1, Rue Guillaume Paradin, Lyon 69372, France.
E-mail address: jacqueline.trouillas@univ-lyon1.fr

Endocrinol Metab Clin N Am 44 (2015) 11–18
http://dx.doi.org/10.1016/j.ecl.2014.10.001
0889-8529/15/$ – see front matter © 2015 Elsevier Inc. All rights reserved.

INTRODUCTION

Endocrine pituitary tumors arise from adenohypophyseal cells. Their classification has evolved over the years supported by continuing improvements of numerous technologies (MRI, electron microscopy [EM], and immunohistochemistry). Indeed, the tinctorial classification of pituitary endocrine tumors into 3 types, acidophilic, basophilic, and chromophobic, was substituted by an IHC classification into 5 types: GH, PRL, ACTH, thyroid-stimulating hormone (TSH), and follicle-stimulating hormone (FSH)-luteinizing hormone (LH), plus a dozen ultrastructural subtypes. Pituitary endocrine tumors are also clinically classified into functioning and nonfunctioning tumors. Although classically considered as benign tumors, recent studies suggest revision of this status. Indeed, 30% to 45% are invasive for the cavernous or the sphenoid sinus.[1] Besides the endocrine signs, because of hormonal hypersecretion or pituitary deficit, clinical and therapeutic management of pituitary tumor growth or invasion is difficult. Some tumors are considered as aggressive, based on their resistance to conventional treatment or recurrence during follow-up.[2] Rare tumors (0.2%), called carcinomas may metastasize and often progress despite multiple treatments.[3–6] The absence of a consensual prognostic classification of pituitary endocrine tumors makes the planning of homogeneous medical strategies hard.

This review stresses the benefits for the clinician of including a detailed pathologic diagnosis when planning the therapeutic management of these patients.

A NEW PRACTICAL PROGNOSTIC CLASSIFICATION FOR CLINICIANS

Recently, the authors proposed a prognostic clinicopathologic classification,[7] which takes into account the tumor size and the IHC subtype (PRL, GH, FSH/LH, ACTH, and TSH). A grading system (grade 1a, noninvasive; 1b, noninvasive and proliferative; 2a, invasive; 2b, invasive and proliferative; and 3, metastatic) (**Table 1**), based on classifications used for other endocrine tumors of the foregut[8] includes both the invasion and proliferation status (**Box 1**). A case-control study of a cohort of 410 patients with at least 8 years follow-up demonstrated its highly significant prognostic value for predicting postoperative disease-free outcome or recurrence/progression status, across all tumors and for each tumor type. Indeed, at 8 years follow-up, an invasive and proliferative tumor (grade 2b) was 25 and 12 times more likely to persist and progress, respectively, than a noninvasive and nonproliferative tumor (grade 1a). These results confirm those obtained in the authors' preliminary study on 94 PRL tumors[9] classified into 3 groups, ie, noninvasive, invasive, and aggressive-invasive, corresponding, respectively, to grades 1a, 2a, and 2b of the new classification.

Table 1 Guide for the establishment of the pituitary tumor grade				
Grade	1a	1b	2a	2b
Invasion	0	0	+	+
Proliferation	0	+	0	+

Invasion: histologic and/or radiological (MRI) signs of cavernous or sphenoid sinus invasion.
 Proliferation: presence of at least 2 of the 3 criteria: mitoses: n greater than 2; Ki-67: greater than or equal to 3%; p53: positive.

Box 1
Clinicopathologic classification of the pituitary endocrine tumors

The classification is based on the following 3 characteristics:

1. Tumor size into micro (<10 mm), macro ($\geq$10 mm), and giant (>40 mm) by MRI

2. Tumor type into GH, PRL, ACTH, FSH/LH, and TSH by immunohistochemistry

3. Tumor grade based on the following criteria:

   Invasion defined as histologic and/or radiological (MRI) signs of cavernous or sphenoid sinus invasion

   Proliferation considered based on the presence of at least 2 of the following 3 criteria:

   Mitoses: n greater than 2 per 10 HPF

   Ki-67: greater than or equal to 3%

   p53: positive (>10 strongly positive nuclei per 10 HPF)

The 5 grades are the following:

Grade 1a: noninvasive tumor

Grade 1b: noninvasive and proliferative tumor

Grade 2a: invasive tumor

Grade 2b: invasive and proliferative tumor

Grade 3: metastatic tumor (cerebrospinal or systemic metastases)

Abbreviation: HPF, high-power field.
   From Trouillas J, Roy P, Sturm N, et al. A new prognostic clinicopathological classification of pituitary adenomas: a multicentric case-control study of 410 patients with 8 years postoperative follow-up. Acta Neuropathol 2013;126(1):127; with permission.

Criteria Used in This Classification

Invasion

Invasion is assessed using MRI, because its histologic proof is rare (9% of invasive tumors in the authors' series). Only invasion into the sphenoid sinus, confirmed by the infiltrated respiratory mucosae on histology, and unequivocal invasion of the cavernous sinus, also appreciable by preoperative endoscopy, are considered. Using multivariate statistical analysis and a receiver operating characteristic curve, the authors found invasion to be a major prognostic factor in predicting both disease-free status after surgical removal[10] and recurrence/progression.[11] So the authors believe that invasion should be added to the recently published synoptic checklist for pituitary lesions.[12] Indeed, pathologists have now an easier access to this criterion through the consultation of surgical and pituitary imaging reports in electronic medical records.

Proliferation

Tumor proliferation was evaluated using Ki-67 index and mitotic count. p53, a well-known tumor suppressor gene, was used as an additional marker of tumor aggressive behavior. Considering the controversial value of these markers, especially Ki-67[11,13,14] and the lack of methodological standards and validated cutoffs for p53 (reviewed in Ref.[15]), the authors defined proliferation as the presence of at least 2 of these 3 markers. Cutoff values were 3% for Ki-67 proliferation index and n greater than 2 mitoses per 10 high-power fields for mitotic count, similar to endocrine pancreatic tumors.[8] The authors evaluated p53 in terms of its positivity.

with 2.5% in the Saeger and colleagues' series.[34] Moreover, it is only a morphologic definition lacking any correlation with postoperative results, progression, and recurrence. As a consequence, one expert questioned whether it is clinically helpful.[35]

Prolactin tumors in men

The larger size of PRL tumors observed in men is often attributed to delayed diagnosis. However, Delgrange and colleagues[36] demonstrated a lack of correlation in either sex between tumor size and age or duration of symptoms. Rather, the PRL tumors in men seemed more often invasive and resistant to dopamine agonists than those in women. An early and aggressive postoperative treatment may thus avoid evolution to carcinoma in such patients.[37]

SUMMARY

Recent advances in pituitary tumor classification now allow the early identification of tumors suspected of malignancy (grade 2b) or pathologic subtypes (silent GH and ACTH tumor or PRL tumor in men) with high risk of recurrence and resistance to conventional treatment strategies. Until markers of malignancy are discovered, comprehensive clinicopathologic classification of pituitary tumors remains the best indicator of clinical behavior in patients, but its suggested prognostic value has to be proved in prospective studies. In such patients, a multidisciplinary approach involving neurosurgeons, endocrinologists, pathologists, and oncologists should allow an optimized therapeutic strategy that takes into account new therapeutic options, in addition to conventional therapies associating somatostatin or dopamine agonist surgery and radiotherapy.

ACKNOWLEDGMENTS

We thank Emily Witty from Angloscribe for help with the English translation; P. Gérardi for typing the article; P Chevallier, A. Reynaud, and M.P. Guigard for technical assistance; as well as all the members of HYPOPRONOS.

REFERENCES

1. Meij BP, Lopes MB, Ellegala DB, et al. The long-term significance of microscopic dural invasion in 354 patients with pituitary adenomas treated with transsphenoidal surgery. J Neurosurg 2002;96(2):195–208.
2. Raverot G, Castinetti F, Jouanneau E, et al. Pituitary carcinomas and aggressive pituitary tumours: merits and pitfalls of temozolomide treatment. Clin Endocrinol 2012;76(6):769–75.
3. Kaltsas GA, Nomikos P, Kontogeorgos G, et al. Diagnosis and management of pituitary carcinomas. J Clin Endocrinol Metab 2005;90(5):3089–99.
4. Dudziak K, Honegger J, Bornemann A, et al. Pituitary carcinoma with malignant growth from first presentation and fulminant clinical course. Case report and review of the literature. J Clin Endocrinol Metab 2011;96(9):2665–9.
5. Jouanneau E, Wierinckx A, Ducray F, et al. New targeted therapies in pituitary carcinoma resistant to temozolomide. Pituitary 2012;15(1):37–43.
6. Raverot G, Sturm N, de Fraipont F, et al. Temozolomide treatment in aggressive pituitary tumors and pituitary carcinomas: a French multicenter experience. J Clin Endocrinol Metab 2010;95(10):4592–9.
7. Trouillas J, Roy P, Sturm N, et al. A new prognostic clinicopathological classification of pituitary adenomas: a multicentric case-control study of 410 patients with 8 years post-operative follow-up. Acta Neuropathol 2013;126(1):123–35.

8. Rindi G, Kloppel G, Alhman H, et al. TNM staging of foregut (neuro)endocrine tumors: a consensus proposal including a grading system. Virchows Arch 2006; 449(4):395–401.
9. Raverot G, Wierinckx A, Dantony E, et al. Prognostic factors in prolactin pituitary tumors: clinical, histological, and molecular data from a series of 94 patients with a long postoperative follow-up. J Clin Endocrinol Metab 2010;95(4):1708–16.
10. Wolfsberger S, Knosp E. Comments on the WHO 2004 classification of pituitary tumors. Acta Neuropathol 2006;111(1):66–7.
11. Righi A, Agati P, Sisto A, et al. A classification tree approach for pituitary adenomas. Hum Pathol 2012;43(10):1627–37.
12. Nose V, Ezzat S, Horvath E, et al. Protocol for the examination of specimens from patients with primary pituitary tumors. Arch Pathol Lab Med 2011;135(5):640–6.
13. Knosp E, Steiner E, Kitz K, et al. Pituitary adenomas with invasion of the cavernous sinus space: a magnetic resonance imaging classification compared with surgical findings. Neurosurgery 1993;33(4):610–7.
14. Thapar K, Kovacs K, Scheithauer BW, et al. Proliferative activity and invasiveness among pituitary adenomas and carcinomas: an analysis using the MIB-1 antibody. Neurosurgery 1996;38(1):99–106.
15. Trouillas J. In search of a prognostic classification of endocrine pituitary tumors. Endocr Pathol 2014;25:124–32.
16. Gurlek A, Karavitaki N, Ansorge O, et al. What are the markers of aggressiveness in prolactinomas? Changes in cell biology, extracellular matrix components, angiogenesis and genetics. Eur J Endocrinol 2007;156(2):143–53.
17. Mete O, Asa SL. Clinicopathological correlations in pituitary adenomas. Brain Pathol 2012;22(4):443–53.
18. Raverot G, Jouanneau E, Trouillas J. Management of endocrine disease: clinicopathological classification and molecular markers of pituitary tumours for personalized therapeutic strategies. Eur J Endocrinol 2014;170(4):R121–32.
19. Scheithauer BW, Kurtkaya-Yapicier O, Kovacs KT, et al. Pituitary carcinoma: a clinicopathological review. Neurosurgery 2005;56(5):1066–74.
20. Wierinckx A, Auger C, Devauchelle P, et al. A diagnostic marker set for invasion, proliferation, and aggressiveness of prolactin pituitary tumors. Endocr Relat Cancer 2007;14(3):887–900.
21. Wierinckx A, Roche M, Raverot G, et al. Integrated genomic profiling identifies loss of chromosome 11p impacting transcriptomic activity in aggressive pituitary PRL tumors. Brain Pathol 2011;21(5):533–43.
22. Lloyd RV, Kovacs K, Young WF Jr, et al. Pituitary tumours: introduction. In chapter 1: tumours of the pituitary. In: DeLellis RA, Lloyd RV, Heitz PU, et al, editors. World Hearth Organization classification of tumours. Lyon (France): IARC Press; 2004. p. 10–3.
23. Obari A, Sano T, Ohyama K, et al. Clinicopathological features of growth hormone-producing pituitary adenomas: difference among various types defined by cytokeratin distribution pattern including a transitional form. Endocr Pathol 2008;19(2):82–91.
24. Fougner SL, Casar-Borota O, Heck A, et al. Adenoma granulation pattern correlates with clinical variables and effect of somatostatin analogue treatment in a large series of patients with acromegaly. Clin Endocrinol 2012;76(1):96–102.
25. Chinezu L, Vasiljevic A, Jouanneau E, et al. Expression of somatostatin receptors, SSTR2A and SSTR5, in 108 endocrine pituitary tumors using immunohistochemical detection with new specific monoclonal antibodies. Hum Pathol 2014;45(1): 71–7.

recent report (2006–2010) from the Central Brain Tumor Registry of the United States indicates that pituitary tumors account for 15.8% of all primary brain/central nervous system tumors, rising to 32% in young adults.[2] Most pituitary adenomas appear to occur sporadically and the molecular genetic abnormalities that exist in the tumor tissue are legion.[3,4] It is difficult to predict generally whether any individual is at risk of developing a pituitary adenoma; conditions in which pituitary adenomas occur as part of a heritable syndrome need to be well recognized clinically so as to allow effective screening and early diagnosis. The most frequent among these conditions are familial isolated pituitary adenoma (FIPA) and multiple endocrine neoplasia type 1 (MEN1), which each account for approximately 2% of pituitary adenomas in general.[5] FIPA occurs in kindreds with 2 or more related individuals affected with pituitary adenomas in the absence of MEN1 or other syndromic causes.[6,7] We identified and characterized this clinical condition from 1999 to 2006, and since then more than 200 kindreds have been identified.[8] To date, one important genetic cause of FIPA has been identified: inactivating mutations in the aryl hydrocarbon receptor interacting protein (AIP) gene.[9,10] Although FIPA is the most frequent clinical presentation of AIP mutations, other significant at-risk populations exist, including young patients with pituitary adenomas. Here we trace the current state of knowledge regarding the clinical features of FIPA and the characteristics of pituitary adenomas due to AIP mutations.

FAMILIAL ISOLATED PITUITARY ADENOMAS

Following a single-center study in 1999, we noted the existence of both acromegaly and nonacromegaly families without MEN1 and other genetic conditions.[6,11] After confirming these findings internationally, the term familial isolated pituitary adenoma (FIPA) was coined to describe this clinical syndrome.[7] FIPA kindreds can present with the same pituitary tumor phenotypes among affected individuals (homogeneous FIPA) or mixtures of different adenomas can occur in the same kindred (heterogeneous FIPA).[7] Overall, FIPA accounts for approximately 2% of pituitary adenomas in our experience.[7] The disease characteristics outlined in **Box 1** can be discerned.[7,8,12]

ARYL HYDROCARBON RECEPTOR INTERACTING PROTEIN GENE MUTATIONS IN PITUITARY ADENOMAS

In 2006, the involvement of the inactivating mutations in the AIP gene in the pathogenesis of pituitary adenomas was discovered.[9] AIP has 6 exons and encodes a 330–amino acid protein that is widely but variably expressed (expression levels are particularly high in pituitary growth hormone (GH) and prolactin-secreting cells). In that study, patients had either acromegaly alone (homogeneous FIPA) or acromegaly plus prolactinomas (heterogeneous FIPA).[9] Some cases had mixed GH and prolactin cells in their tumor samples, which explains the frequent combined GH/prolactin co-secretion in these cases.[10,13] The R304 residue also appears to be a hot spot for mutations, as mutations (p.R304X/Q) have been seen in a variety of different populations de novo.[8] Similarly, common mutations, such as the missense p.R271W mutation, have been seen in geographically diverse and unrelated kindreds across the globe.[8,10,14]

In the time since the initial discovery of AIP, many studies have been performed in general and in specific populations. Extensive testing among unselected patients with pituitary adenoma with apparently sporadic tumors revealed a low rate of AIP

Box 1
Characteristics of FIPA

FIPA families can be either homogeneous (60%) or heterogeneous (40%) in terms of the pituitary adenoma type that occurs in the kindred. All general types of secreting and nonsecreting pituitary adenomas have been reported in FIPA.

Homogeneous FIPA is composed of mainly acromegaly (58%), prolactinoma (32%), and nonfunctioning adenoma families (7%); rare Cushing disease families also exist.

Heterogeneous FIPA has a broad profile consisting of prolactinomas in combination with acromegaly, nonfunctioning adenomas, and others in 78% of cases. The most frequent heterogeneous FIPA phenotype is a combination of acromegaly and prolactinomas in affected members (42%).

Taking the tumor types from all FIPA families together and comparing them with the general prevalence of different pituitary tumors in the general population, it can be seen that although prolactinomas are the most frequent tumor type in FIPA (38%), the frequency is much lower than in the general population (66%). This is partially because of the high prevalence of somatotropinomas in FIPA (35%) as compared with general epidemiologic data (13%–15%).

Most cases involve first-degree relationships among the affected members within the kindred.

Affected members within kindreds can number between 2 and 8 cases with pituitary adenomas; most families have 2 to 3 cases with adenomas.

Patients with FIPA have earlier disease onset as compared with non-FIPA cases, being diagnosed 4 years earlier. In multigenerational FIPA families, patients in the younger generations are diagnosed up to 20 years earlier than their forebears.

In homogeneous somatotropinoma families, the disease onset is young and tumors are likely to be large and invasive (the rate of *AIP* mutations in such families contributes significantly to this pattern of tumor behavior.

Nonfunctioning pituitary adenomas and prolactinomas occurring in the setting of heterogeneous FIPA families are more likely to be large and invasive than non-FIPA tumor counterparts.

---

mutations (2%–3%). Hence, widespread screening of unselected populations is unlikely to be useful.

THE ROLE OF ARYL HYDROCARBON RECEPTOR INTERACTING PROTEIN MUTATIONS IN FAMILIAL ISOLATED PITUITARY ADENOMAS

We initially studied 73 FIPA families and found approximately 20% of families were affected with *AIP* mutations[10]; a mutation rate of approximately 20% remains valid.[8] Affected families had acromegaly, prolactinomas and nonsecreting pituitary adenomas. The negative results of screening studies for other genes suggest that other genetic causes for FIPA remain to be discovered.[15] *AIP* mutations have been seen in both homogeneous and heterogeneous FIPA kindreds, although there appears to be a tendency for *AIP* to associate with families with somatotropinomas. A novel presentation of *AIP*-mutation–positive FIPA is that of pituitary apoplexy, which has been reported as an acute or late presentation.[16–18]

ROLE OF ARYL HYDROCARBON RECEPTOR INTERACTING PROTEIN MUTATIONS IN YOUNG PATIENTS WITH PITUITARY ADENOMA

Young age at disease onset is characteristic of *AIP* mutation cases. Almost all *AIP* mutation–positive cases were diagnosed before the age of 40, and most were far younger. Among FIPA cases, patients with *AIP* mutations are statistically significantly younger than cases from FIPA families that do not have *AIP* mutations.[10,12,17] Based on those results, targeted studies in young patient populations have been performed. In our series of patients with the National Institutes of Health, among pediatric patients with Cushing disease, *AIP* positivity was low (1.4%); the rate was higher when pediatric somatotropinomas and syndromic cases were included (4.5%).[19] We studied 163 patients with sporadic pituitary macroadenoma aged younger than 30 years at disease onset; 11.7% had *AIP* mutations.[20] Combining macroadenoma with an age younger than 18 at disease onset led to a very high rate of *AIP* mutation identification of 20.5% of cases.[20] This high rate is similar to that seen when large sporadic series are filtered for age at diagnosis of younger than 18.[21,22]

OVERVIEW OF ARYL HYDROCARBON RECEPTOR INTERACTING PROTEIN IN PITUITARY ADENOMAS

AIP mutations are now established as one of the few germline causes of pituitary adenoma. A synthesis of the current literature indicates that various types of mutations and deletions of *AIP* can underlie pituitary adenoma pathogenesis.[8,23] In a recent overview of the published literature, 132 (70.2%) of 215 *AIP* mutation/deletion–associated cases were somatotrope/somatolactotrope adenomas, 13.5% were prolactinomas, 6% were nonfunctioning adenomas, and 1.9% were Cushing disease.[8] Other tumor types, such as thyroid-stimulating hormone secreting adenomas, are very rarely associated with *AIP* mutations. The general characteristics of *AIP* mutation cases are shown in **Box 2**.

Box 2
Clinical characteristics of *AIP* mutation–related pituitary adenomas

Predominantly male (61%)

Predominantly macroadenomas at diagnosis (88%) with extrasellar extension

FIPA is the most common presentation (68%)

Mainly acromegaly or prolactinomas (84%)

Young age at diagnosis (78% aged <30 years)

First symptoms frequently occur in childhood or adolescence

Gigantism is particularly frequent (36%)

Somatostatin analog resistance is characteristic in acromegaly cases (**Fig. 1**); prolactinomas may require surgery

Multimodal therapy often required to bring about disease control

Apoplexy may be a feature

Most cases identified by sequencing; multiplex ligation-dependent probe amplification analysis for deletions useful for suspicious cases (with the other clinical features outlined in the Box) that are normal for *AIP* on sequencing

AIP mutations in families have a low penetrance (20%), and most mutation carriers never develop an adenoma. Conversely generation skipping can occur between affected members with *AIP* mutations and pituitary adenomas, making familial awareness of the condition important to early diagnosis.

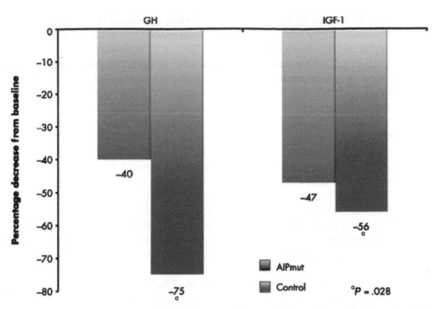

Fig. 1. Resistance to somatostatin analogs is evidenced by smaller reductions in GH and insulinlike growth factor-1 (IGF-1) in *AIP* mutation-related somatotropinomas (AIPmut) (n = 75) versus controls matched for age and sex (n = 232). (*From* Beckers A, Aaltonen LA, Daly AF, et al. Familial isolated pituitary adenomas (FIPA) and the pituitary adenoma predisposition due to mutations in the aryl hydrocarbon receptor interacting protein (AIP) gene. Endocr Rev 2013;34:254; with permission.)

SUMMARY

FIPA is an evolving clinical syndrome of isolated pituitary adenomas with multiple clinical patterns of presentation and behavior. This diversity suggests that many different pathophysiological processes are at work. Among FIPA families, mutations or deletions of *AIP* are an important cause, which can be studied in screening of targeted groups of patients, which is not only limited to FIPA itself. Young patients, particularly children and adolescents with somatotropinomas or prolactinomas, warrant consideration for *AIP* screening. In addition, young adults with macroadenomas or with gigantism are an enriched population for *AIP* testing. Ideally, this type of genetic screening of affected cases should be done in parallel with other genes as part of an integrated testing system. The pairing of *AIP* and MEN1 testing in young patients with aggressive adenomas has proven itself to be an efficient method to identify affected cases.[24] However, data suggest that widespread unfocussed screening of large patient populations with pituitary adenomas is unlikely to yield a large number of positive cases and such studies are unlikely to have scientific benefit. In FIPA families with *AIP* mutations, penetrance is low, in the region of 20%.[8] For this reason, genetic counseling is important to allow for proper explanations of the likelihood of developing a pituitary tumor in those carrying an *AIP* mutation.

REFERENCES

1. Daly AF, Rixhon M, Adam C, et al. High prevalence of pituitary adenomas: a cross-sectional study in the province of Liege, Belgium. J Clin Endocrinol Metab 2006;91:4769–75.

caused by head trauma or irradiation. At the other extreme is acromegaly, which is an excess of GH secretion, usually caused by a pituitary adenoma. If acromegaly starts before puberty, it can result in a giant phenotype. Adult acromegaly has a less prominent phenotype because the excess growth focuses on extremities and internal organs. Nevertheless, the condition is associated with increased morbidity and mortality if left untreated.

Accurate measurement of GH and IGF-I is crucial for diagnosis and monitoring of the disorders of the GH–IGF-I axis. For each of these hormones, there are multiple steps where the reliability of the laboratory analyses can be affected. A classic paper from 2007 had the same GH sample measured in 104 centers and an IGF-I sample in 23 centers across the UK using variable assay methods. The results varied more than 3-fold for GH and up to 2.5-fold for IGF-I.[1] Clearly, choosing an established and reliable assay method is highly important, but not enough if there are problems with sampling conditions or determining appropriate cutoffs for making a correct diagnosis. The aim of this review is to introduce the potential pitfalls in GH and IGF-I measurements and to help avoid them. Regarding assay design, we focus on immunoassays even though biological assays that evaluate the biological activity of GH and IGF-I also exist.[2–4] However, because the biological assays depend on activation, proliferation, or differentiation of living cells, their reproducibility is not good enough for routine clinical purposes.

GROWTH HORMONE

GH is a rather stable protein and does not require more than standard care during sample processing. Total GH as well as the different GH isoforms exhibit a remarkable preanalytical stability.[5] Furthermore, a recent study demonstrated that 22 kD GH concentrations as measured by an immunoassay did not change over a period of more than 10 years when samples were stored at −80°C.[6] Traditionally, the preferred matrix to measure GH is serum, but most of the currently available assays can also be used with plasma samples. Even though GH sample handling is easy, there are plenty of other factors that make measuring GH and interpreting measured GH concentrations a challenge. First, the biology of GH secretion is complex: circulating GH concentrations depend highly on when, how, and of whom GH is measured. GH is secreted in a pulsatile manner and the magnitude of pulses follows a circadian pattern. Furthermore, nutritional status, exercise, sleep, stress, and body temperature all affect GH levels, additionally contributing to the high intraindividual variation in GH levels. Therefore, a stimulation or suppression test is used to obtain peak or nadir GH values, which then are used for diagnosis. Age has a major impact on GH levels; GH levels peak at late adolescence and decline from age 20 such that only very low levels can be detected at and after age 60.[7] Additionally, women have two to three times higher mean GH levels than men do.[8] In the current obesity epidemic, one has to also take into account the effects of body mass index (BMI) on GH levels; obese individuals have lower GH secretion as well as faster GH clearance rates.[9,10] Abdominal fat is also a negative regulator of GH and is correlated with decreased GH levels, even in individuals with normal BMI.[11]

In general, a stimulation test and a following peak GH value are used for diagnosis of GH deficiency and a suppression test with GH nadir is applied when diagnosing acromegaly. There are several validated GH stimulation tests, such as the traditional insulin tolerance test, but the use of GH-releasing hormone in combination with arginine, which inhibits somatostatin, is suggested to provide the most accurate results in children as well as adults.[12,13] For the GH-releasing hormone + arginine test,

BMI-specific (<25, 25–30, and >30 kg/m^2) cutoffs have been determined.[14] The standard test to diagnose excess GH secretion as in acromegaly is an oral glucose tolerance test. Care has to be taken when interpreting results from these provocative tests. There is considerable variation in the cutoffs for GH stimulation tests set by different medical societies,[15] even though assay-specific cutoffs are recommended.[13,14] Unfortunately, published and well-validated data are only available for selected assay systems and testing conditions.[13,16–18] Regarding the suppression test, the increased assay sensitivity as well as the change in assay calibration has taken the GH nadir indicating control of acromegaly from less than 2.5 µg/L[19] to less than 0.4 µg/L.[14]

GH is present in circulation in several different isoforms and isomers. The most common GH variant is the 22 kD GH, also known as GH-1 or GH-N, secreted from anterior pituitary. The pituitary produces also smaller GH molecules, such as the 20 kD GH variant, as result of alternative gene splicing. The 20 kD isoform displays longer half-life but lower potency than 22 kD GH. In circulation, homodimerization and heterodimerization of these molecules adds to the variety of the GH isoforms present.[20] Under normal conditions as well as in response to a variety of stimuli, the different isoforms of GH are secreted in parallel.[20,21] It has been speculated that the proportion of non–22 kD GH isoforms may be increased in acromegaly,[22,23] but this increase is not likely to be large enough to lead to misdiagnosis even when using 22 kD-specific GH assays, and no relationship between specific isoforms and types of disease has been shown. The only exception is during pregnancy, when a placental GH (GH-2 or GH-V) replaces pituitary GH.[24] To avoid problems with monitoring acromegaly during gestation, the GH assay being used in such a situation should be tested for pregnancy serum interference.[25] Another molecule that can cause problems for monitoring acromegaly is the GH receptor antagonist drug pegvisomant, which closely resembles pituitary GH. Literature only reports few GH assays that are free of pegvisomant interference, whereas most investigated assays greatly overestimate or underestimate GH levels in presence of pegvisomant.[26]

"Go permissive or go specific?" is a traditional question when designing an assay for GH. The use of polyclonal antibodies allows detection of several GH isoforms, whereas monoclonal antibodies only bind to a specific molecular form of GH. The current consensus is to "go specific" because no disease is known that only affects a single isoform, and assay standardization and comparability as well as harmonization of cutoff values are considered more important than measurement of multiple GH isoforms.[27] The recommendation is to limit detection to the 22 kD pituitary GH, which also means that cross-reactivity to other GH isoforms should be investigated and made available. Other molecules that are similar to GH and therefore potential cross-reactants include the other members of the GH gene family, that is, placental GH and placental lactogens, as well as prolactin.

Limiting GH assays to measure the 22 kD pituitary isoform is not enough to harmonize GH assays. Another major source of variability between different assays is the use of different standard preparations for calibration of GH immunoassays. A further source of confusion in the past was that some laboratories reported GH concentrations in activity (mU/L), whereas others used mass units (µg/L). The existence of various conversion factors between the 2 added to the confusion. Currently, all GH assays should be calibrated to the international reference standard 98/574 (National Institute for Biological Standards and Control), a recombinant pituitary GH preparation of high purity,[27] and all GH concentrations should be measured and reported in mass units.

Finally, adding to the diversity of GH isoforms in circulation, GH also forms complexes with GH binding protein (GHBP), to which approximately 50% of circulating thoroughly validated, and where all the relevant information about cross-reactivity and normative data is disclosed and published in peer-reviewed journals. This is the only way to increase transparency for laboratories and clinicians and to allow meaningful interpretation of laboratory results.

REFERENCES

1. Pokrajac A, Wark G, Ellis AR, et al. Variation in GH and IGF-I assays limits the applicability of international consensus criteria to local practice. Clin Endocrinol (Oxf) 2007;67(1):65–70.
2. Juárez-Aguilar E, Castro-Muñozledo F, Kuri-Harcuch W. A simple and sensitive assay for GH activity based on 3T3-F442A cell differentiation. Biochem Biophys Res Commun 2003;311(4):935–41.
3. Tanaka T, Shiu RP, Gout PW, et al. A new sensitive and specific bioassay for lactogenic hormones: measurement of prolactin and growth hormone in human serum. J Clin Endocrinol Metab 1980;51(5):1058–63.
4. Chen JW, Ledet T, Orskov H, et al. A highly sensitive and specific assay for determination of IGF-I bioactivity in human serum. Am J Physiol Endocrinol Metab 2003;284(6):E1149–55.
5. Bidlingmaier M, Suhr J, Ernst A, et al. High-sensitivity chemiluminescence immunoassays for detection of growth hormone doping in sports. Clin Chem 2009; 55(3):445–53.
6. Wagner IV, Paetzold C, Gausche R, et al. Clinical evidence-based cutoff limits for GH stimulation tests in children with a backup of results with reference to mass spectrometry. Eur J Endocrinol 2014;171(3):389–97.
7. Zadik Z, Chalew SA, McCarter RJ Jr, et al. The influence of age on the 24-hour integrated concentration of growth hormone in normal individuals. J Clin Endocrinol Metab 1985;60(3):513–6.
8. van den Berg G, Veldhuis JD, Frölich M, et al. An amplitude-specific divergence in the pulsatile mode of growth hormone (GH) secretion underlies the gender difference in mean GH concentrations in men and premenopausal women. J Clin Endocrinol Metab 1996;81(7):2460–7.
9. Veldhuis JD, Iranmanesh A, Ho KK, et al. Dual defects in pulsatile growth hormone secretion and clearance subserve the hyposomatotropism of obesity in man. J Clin Endocrinol Metab 1991;72(1):51–9.
10. Langendonk JG, Meinders AE, Burggraaf J, et al. Influence of obesity and body fat distribution on growth hormone kinetics in humans. Am J Physiol 1999;277(5 Pt 1):E824–9.
11. Vahl N, Jørgensen JO, Skjaerbaek C, et al. Abdominal adiposity rather than age and sex predicts mass and regularity of GH secretion in healthy adults. Am J Physiol 1997;272(6 Pt 1):E1108–16.
12. Ghigo E, Bellone J, Aimaretti G, et al. Reliability of provocative tests to assess growth hormone secretory status. Study in 472 normally growing children. J Clin Endocrinol Metab 1996;81(9):3323–7.
13. Markkanen HM, Pekkarinen T, Välimäki MJ, et al. Comparison of two growth hormone stimulation tests and their cut-off limits in healthy adults at an outpatient clinic. Growth Horm IGF Res 2013;23(5):165–9.
14. Ho KK, 2007 GH Deficiency Consensus Workshop Participants. Consensus guidelines for the diagnosis and treatment of adults with GH deficiency II: a statement of the GH Research Society in association with the European Society for Pediatric Endocrinology, Lawson Wilkins Society, European Society of Endocrinology,

Japan Endocrine Society, and Endocrine Society of Australia. Eur J Endocrinol 2007;157(6):695–700.

15. Bogazzi F, Manetti L, Lombardi M, et al. Impact of different cut-off limits of peak GH after GHRH-arginine stimulatory test, single IGF1 measurement, or their combination in identifying adult patients with GH deficiency. Eur J Endocrinol 2011; 164(5):685–93.

16. Binder G, Huller E, Blumenstock G, et al. Auxology-based cut-off values for biochemical testing of GH secretion in childhood. Growth Horm IGF Res 2011; 21(4):212–8.

17. Chaler EA, Ballerini GA, Lazzati JM, et al. Cut-off values of serum growth hormone (GH) in pharmacological stimulation tests (PhT) evaluated in short-statured children using a chemiluminescent immunometric assay (ICMA) calibrated with the International Recombinant Human GH Standard 98/574. Clin Chem Lab Med 2013;51(5):e95–7.

18. Klose M, Stochholm K, Janukonyté J, et al. Prevalence of posttraumatic growth hormone deficiency is highly dependent on the diagnostic set-up: results from The Danish National Study on Posttraumatic Hypopituitarism. J Clin Endocrinol Metab 2014;99(1):101–10.

19. Bidlingmaier M, Strasburger CJ. What endocrinologists should know about growth hormone measurements. Endocrinol Metab Clin North Am 2007;36(1):101–8.

20. Baumann GP. Growth hormone isoforms. Growth Horm IGF Res 2009;19(4): 333–40.

21. Tong J, D'Alessio D, Ramisch J, et al. Ghrelin stimulation of growth hormone isoforms: parallel secretion of total and 20-kDa growth hormone and relation to insulin sensitivity in healthy humans. J Clin Endocrinol Metab 2012;97(9):3366–74.

22. Boguszewski CL, Johannsson G, Bengtsson BA, et al. Circulating non-22-kilodalton growth hormone isoforms in acromegalic men before and after transsphenoidal surgery. J Clin Endocrinol Metab 1997;82(5):1516–21.

23. Lima GA, Wu Z, Silva CM, et al. Growth hormone isoforms in acromegalic patients before and after treatment with octreotide LAR. Growth Horm IGF Res 2010;20(2): 87–92.

24. Wu Z, Bidlingmaier M, Friess SC, et al. A new nonisotopic, highly sensitive assay for the measurement of human placental growth hormone: development and clinical implications. J Clin Endocrinol Metab 2003;88(2):804–11.

25. Dias ML, Vieira JG, Abucham J. Detecting and solving the interference of pregnancy serum, in a GH immunometric assay. Growth Horm IGF Res 2013;23(1–2):13–8.

26. Manolopoulou J, Alami Y, Petersenn S, et al. Automated 22-kD growth hormone-specific assay without interference from Pegvisomant. Clin Chem 2012;58(10): 1446–56.

27. Clemmons DR. Consensus statement on the standardization and evaluation of growth hormone and insulin-like growth factor assays. Clin Chem 2011;57(4):555–9.

28. Milani D, Carmichael JD, Welkowitz J, et al. Variability and reliability of single serum IGF-I measurements: impact on determining predictability of risk ratios in disease development. J Clin Endocrinol Metab 2004;89(5):2271–4.

29. Nguyen TV, Nelson AE, Howe CJ, et al. Within-subject variability and analytic imprecision of insulinlike growth factor axis and collagen markers: implications for clinical diagnosis and doping tests. Clin Chem 2008;54(8):1268–76.

30. Erotokritou-Mulligan I, Eryl Bassett E, Cowan DA, et al. The use of growth hormone (GH)-dependent markers in the detection of GH abuse in sport: physiological intra-individual variation of IGF-I, type 3 pro-collagen (P-III-P) and the GH-2000 detection score. Clin Endocrinol (Oxf) 2010;72(4):520–6.

31. Borofsky ND, Vogelman JH, Krajcik RA, et al. Utility of insulin-like growth factor-1 as a biomarker in epidemiologic studies. Clin Chem 2002;48(12):2248–51.
32. Bancos I, Algeciras-Schimnich A, Grebe SK, et al. Evaluation of variables influencing the measurement of insulin-like growth factor-1. Endocr Pract 2014; 20(5):421–6.
33. Brabant G, von zur Mühlen A, Wüster C, et al. Serum insulin-like growth factor I reference values for an automated chemiluminescence immunoassay system: results from a multicenter study. Horm Res 2003;60(2):53–60.
34. Bidlingmaier M, Friedrich N, Emeny RT, et al. Reference intervals for insulin-like growth factor-1 (IGF-I) from birth to senescence: results from a multicenter study using a new automated chemiluminescence IGF-I immunoassay conforming to recent international recommendations. J Clin Endocrinol Metab 2014;99(5): 1712–21.
35. Schneider HJ, Saller B, Klotsche J, et al. Opposite associations of age-dependent insulin-like growth factor-I standard deviation scores with nutritional state in normal weight and obese subjects. Eur J Endocrinol 2006;154(5):699–706.
36. Frystyk J, Freda P, Clemmons DR. The current status of IGF-I assays–a 2009 update. Growth Horm IGF Res 2010;20(1):8–18.
37. Gleeson HK, Lissett CA, Shalet SM. Insulin-like growth factor-I response to a single bolus of growth hormone is increased in obesity. J Clin Endocrinol Metab 2005;90(2):1061–7.
38. Renehan AG, Jones J, O'Dwyer ST, et al. Determination of IGF-I, IGF-II, IGFBP-2, and IGFBP-3 levels in serum and plasma: comparisons using the Bland-Altman method. Growth Horm IGF Res 2003;13(6):341–6.
39. Støving RK, Chen JW, Glintborg D, et al. Bioactive insulin-like growth factor (IGF) I and IGF-binding protein-1 in anorexia nervosa. J Clin Endocrinol Metab 2007; 92(6):2323–9.
40. Friedrich N, Wolthers OD, Arafat AM, et al. Age- and sex-specific reference intervals across life span for insulin-like growth factor binding protein 3 (IGFBP-3) and the IGF-I to IGFBP-3 ratio measured by new automated chemiluminescence assays. J Clin Endocrinol Metab 2014;99(5):1675–86.
41. Krebs A, Wallaschofski H, Spilcke-Liss E, et al. Five commercially available insulin-like growth factor I (IGF-I) assays in comparison to the former Nichols Advantage IGF-I in a growth hormone treated population. Clin Chem Lab Med 2008;46(12):1776–83.
42. Cowan DA, Bartlett C. Laboratory issues in the implementation of the marker method. Growth Horm IGF Res 2009;19(4):357–60.
43. Burns C, Rigsby P, Moore M, et al. The First International Standard For Insulin-like Growth Factor-1 (IGF-1) for immunoassay: preparation and calibration in an international collaborative study. Growth Horm IGF Res 2009;19(5):457–62.
44. Cox HD, Lopes F, Woldemariam GA, et al. Interlaboratory agreement of insulin-like growth factor 1 concentrations measured by mass spectrometry. Clin Chem 2014;60(3):541–8.
45. Wieringa GE, Sturgeon CM, Trainer PJ. The harmonisation of growth hormone measurements: taking the next steps. Clin Chim Acta 2014;432:68–71.

Pharmacotherapy for Acromegaly

Future Role for Pasireotide?

Anat Ben-Shlomo, MD

KEYWORDS

- Pharmacotherapy • Acromegaly • Somatostatin receptor ligand • Pasireotide

KEY POINTS

- Pasireotide (SOM230), a new somatostatin receptor ligand with binding affinity to somatostatin receptor subtype 5 (SST5)>SST2>SST3>SST1, has been in clinical trials for the treatment of acromegaly.
- Suppression of growth hormone level to less than 2.5 ng/mL and normalization of insulinlike growth factor I level by pasireotide occurs in one-third of patients with acromegaly.
- Some octreotide-resistant patients respond to pasireotide.
- Pasireotide treatment frequently causes hyperglycemia and diabetes mellitus.

A plethora of literature and guidelines on acromegaly has recently been published. The medical approach to a patient with acromegaly should be guided by clinical symptoms, associated comorbidities, growth hormone (GH) and insulinlike growth factor I (IGF-I) levels, and tumor characteristics.[1] Recent consensus articles have comprehensively summarized medical treatment approach[2]; criteria for cure, including assay pitfalls[3]; and diagnosis and treatment of acromegaly complications.[1]

GH and age-matched IGF-I measurements are most important for the diagnosis and monitoring of acromegaly treatment.[3] Diagnosis is confirmed if random GH levels are greater than 1 ng/mL, nadir GH levels during oral glucose tolerance test (OGTT) are greater than or equal to 0.4 ng/mL, and age-matched IGF-I level is increased. Disease control is determined when random GH levels are less than 1 ng/mL or less than 0.4 ng/mL if measured with a sensitive assay (when treated with somatostatin analogues) or nadir GH level after OGTT is less than 0.4 ng/mL (after surgery) and age-matched IGF-I level is normalized. Only IGF-I levels should be assessed to monitor efficacy of pegvisomant treatment.[1–3]

Disclosure: The author is a consultant to, and received a preclinical grant CSOM230BUS13T from, Novartis.

Pituitary Center, Endocrinology, Diabetes and Metabolism Division, Department of Medicine, Cedars Sinai Medical Center, 8700 Beverly Boulevard, Davis 3066, Los Angeles, CA 90048, USA
E-mail address: benshlomoa@cshs.org

The treatment of choice for acromegaly is surgical removal of the pituitary adenoma the tumor is considered resectable and the surgery is performed by an experienced surgeon.[4] Medical monotherapy is usually used when surgery fails to cure the disease, in patients with an unresectable tumor or who choose not to undergo surgery,[4] and occasionally as primary treatment of treatment-naive patients before surgery.[5]

Pharmacotherapy that has been clinically approved for acromegaly[4] includes somatostatin receptor ligands (SRL; octreotide and lanreotide), pegvisomant, and dopamine agonists. In resistant patients, combination therapy had been proved beneficial, including SRL with dopamine agonist,[6] SRL with pegvisomant,[7] dopamine agonist and pegvisomant,[8] and the addition of estrogens.[4]

Recent published preclinical and clinical trials introduced pasireotide (SOM230; a new pan SRL that is not yet approved by the US Food and Drug Administration and that binds SST5>SSTR2>SSTR3>SST1[9]) as a possible acromegaly treatment. Pasireotide, like octreotide and lanreotide, can be delivered as a short-acting compound injected subcutaneously twice daily or as a long-acting formula (pasireotide LAR) injected intramuscularly every 28 days, and both have been tested in clinical trials for the treatment of acromegaly. The results of the published clinical trials are presented in **Tables 1** and **2**.

A moderate advantage of pasireotide compared with octreotide in treating patients has been suggested. A lower percentage of full responders (random GH <2.5 ng/mL and normalized IGF-I level) to octreotide was reported in the pasireotide studies compared with the previous octreotide and lanreotide studies. A recent meta-analysis of 90 studies (1987–2012) assessing GH and IGF-I response to octreotide LAR or lanreotide Autogel showed that 56% ± 19.7% of patients achieved GH control (using different GH cutoffs, mostly ≤2.5 ng/mL) and 55% ± 17.3% achieved IGF-I normalization.[10] Another study assessing response rate to octreotide LAR in a tertiary center between 2003 and 2012 showed that ~35% of patients achieve control, defined by GH level less than 2.5 ng/mL and IGF-I level less than 1.2 times the upper limit of normal, and only 23% of patients achieved control if a lower threshold level of GH less than 1 ng/mL was used.[11] In the Sandostatin LAR Depot prescribing information brochure the results of 3 clinical trials are cited, showing that 42% to 57% of patients fully respond to Sandostatin LAR if GH level is less than 2.5 ng/mL and normalized IGF-I criteria are used, and only 11% to 22% if GH level is less than 1 ng/mL and normalized IGF-I criteria are used (http://www.accessdata.fda.gov/drugsatfda_docs/label/2006/021008s018s019lbl.pdf). These studies used dosages of between 20 and 40 mg every 28 days and analyzed GH and IGF-I levels after 12 to 28 injections. In contrast with previous reports, and because criteria for cure/remission are stricter, fewer patients with acromegaly achieve control using more rigorous end points, with octreotide or lanreotide treatment.

A phase II randomized, multicenter, open-label, 3-way, crossover core clinical trial studied patients with acromegaly who received octreotide 100 µg subcutaneously 3 times daily for 28 days then immediately switched to pasireotide 200, 400, or 600 µg subcutaneously in random twice daily for 28 days up to 84 days in total.[12] Fifty-eight patients received at least 1 dose of pasireotide and 51 had GH and IGF-I levels measured at the end of the study. Full biochemical response (GH ≤2.5 ng/mL and normalized age-matched and sex-matched IGF-I) was achieved in 27% (14 of 51 patients) and 39% (20 of 51 patients) had tumor volume reduction greater than or equal to 20%. Patients reported a reduction in headaches, fatigue, perspiration, and paresthesia. Although pharmacokinetics were proportional to pasireotide dose, a similar number of full responders was observed in all 3 dose groups; however, plasma pasireotide concentration in responders was higher than in nonresponders.

Table 1
Pasireotide efficacy in patients with acromegaly. Phase II multicenter, open-label clinical trials

| Factors Assessed | Core Study — Octreotide 300 μg Daily, SC, 28 d, Followed by Pasireotide 400/800/1200 μg SC Daily | | Extension Study — Octreotide 300 μg Daily, SC, 28 d, Followed by Pasireotide 400–1800 μg SC Daily | | |
| | 28 d | 84 d | 6 mo | 24 mo | Last Assessment |
	% (n/total)		% (n/total)		
Biochemistry					
GH <2.5 ng/mL and normalized IGF-I	19 (11/58)	27 (14/51)	23 (6/26)	33 (3/9)	N/A
GH <2.5 ng/mL	40 (23/58)	49 (25/51)	46 (12/26)	56 (5/9)	N/A
Normalized IGF-I	26 (15/58)	38 (20/53)	50 (13/26)	56 (5/9)	N/A
Tumor volume					
≥20% reduction	N/A	39 (20/51)	N/A	N/A	59 (17/29)
≥20% increase	N/A	0	N/A	N/A	0
Clinical improvement	Yes	Yes	Yes	Yes	—

Dosing holiday period 43.6 d (range 12–220 d)

Abbreviation: SC, subcutaneously.
Data from Petersenn S, Schopohl J, Barkan A, et al. Pasireotide (SOM230) demonstrates efficacy and safety in patients with acromegaly: a randomized, multicenter, phase II trial. J Clin Endocrinol Metab 2010;95(6):2781–9; and Petersenn S, Farrall AJ, De Block C, et al. Long-term efficacy and safety of subcutaneous pasireotide in acromegaly: results from an open-ended, multicenter, phase II extension study. Pituitary 2014;17(2):132–40.

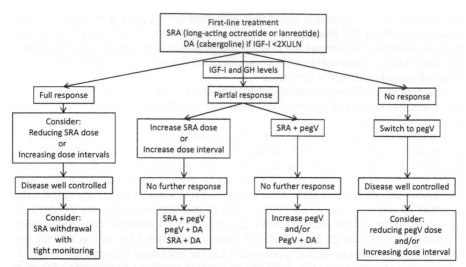

Fig. 1. Recommended pharmacotherapy management of patients with acromegaly. DA, dopamine agonist; pegV, pegvisomant; SRA, somatostatin receptor agonists; ULN, upper limit of normal. (*Adapted from* Giustina A, Chanson P, Kleinberg D, et al. Expert consensus document: a consensus on the medical treatment of acromegaly. Nat Rev Endocrinol 2014;10(4):245; with permission.)

compared with octreotide. Approximately 50% and 19% of patients treated with pasireotide LAR developed hyperglycemia and diabetes mellitus, respectively, compared with 8% and 4% of patients treated with octreotide LAR. Moreover, hyperglycemia was the most common reason for dropping out of the pasireotide LAR treatment arm; Common Terminology Criteria (CTC) grade 3 or 4 hyperglycemia was reported in 9% of patients on pasireotide LAR (1.7% in the octreotide LAR group). Antidiabetic medications were administered to 44.4% of patients treated with pasireotide LAR versus 26.1% of patients treated with octreotide LAR.[15] A recent 24-week analysis of patients with acromegaly treated with pasireotide showed that fasting glucose pretreatment levels greater than 100 mg/dL predicted higher fasting glucose and/or hemoglobin A1c levels with pasireotide treatment. Glucose levels increased immediately on treatment initiation and plateaued with continuous treatment.[19]

In summary, if approved for clinical use in patients with acromegaly, the role of pasireotide in the acromegaly consensus medical flow chart (**Fig. 1**) should be considered. Pasireotide can likely be used for patients with suboptimal response or resistance to treatment with the approved maximal doses of octreotide LAR or lanreotide Autogel. However, the higher frequency of diabetes mellitus is of concern because it is associated with multiple comorbidities, increased mortality, and more frequent medical intervention.

REFERENCES

1. Melmed S, Casanueva FF, Klibanski A, et al. A consensus on the diagnosis and treatment of acromegaly complications. Pituitary 2013;16(3):294–302.
2. Giustina A, Chanson P, Kleinberg D, et al. Expert consensus document: a consensus on the medical treatment of acromegaly. Nat Rev Endocrinol 2014; 10(4):243–8.
3. Giustina A, Chanson P, Bronstein MD, et al. A consensus on criteria for cure of acromegaly. J Clin Endocrinol Metab 2010;95(7):3141–8.

4. Korytnaya E, Barkan A. Pharmacological treatment of acromegaly: its place in the overall therapeutic approach. J Neurooncol 2014;117(3):415–20.
5. Pita-Gutierrez F, Pertega-Diaz S, Pita-Fernandez S, et al. Place of preoperative treatment of acromegaly with somatostatin analog on surgical outcome: a systematic review and meta-analysis. PLoS One 2013;8(4):e61523.
6. Cozzi R, Attanasio R, Lodrini S, et al. Cabergoline addition to depot somatostatin analogues in resistant acromegalic patients: efficacy and lack of predictive value of prolactin status. Clin Endocrinol 2004;61(2):209–15.
7. Neggers SJ, van der Lely AJ. Combination treatment with somatostatin analogues and pegvisomant in acromegaly. Growth Horm IGF Res 2011;21(3): 129–33.
8. Higham CE, Atkinson AB, Aylwin S, et al. Effective combination treatment with cabergoline and low-dose pegvisomant in active acromegaly: a prospective clinical trial. J Clin Endocrinol Metab 2012;97(4):1187–93.
9. Bruns C, Lewis I, Briner U, et al. SOM230: a novel somatostatin peptidomimetic with broad somatotropin release inhibiting factor (SRIF) receptor binding and a unique antisecretory profile. Eur J Endocrinol 2002;146(5):707–16.
10. Carmichael JD, Bonert VS, Nuno M, et al. Acromegaly clinical trial methodology impact on reported biochemical efficacy rates of somatostatin receptor ligand treatments: a meta-analysis. J Clin Endocrinol Metab 2014;99(5):1825–33.
11. Espinosa-de-Los-Monteros AL, Gonzalez B, Vargas G, et al. Octreotide LAR treatment of acromegaly in "real life": long-term outcome at a tertiary care center. Pituitary 2014.
12. Petersenn S, Schopohl J, Barkan A, et al. Pasireotide (SOM230) demonstrates efficacy and safety in patients with acromegaly: a randomized, multicenter, phase II trial. J Clin Endocrinol Metab 2010;95(6):2781–9.
13. Petersenn S, Farrall AJ, De Block C, et al. Long-term efficacy and safety of subcutaneous pasireotide in acromegaly: results from an open-ended, multi-center, Phase II extension study. Pituitary 2014;17(2):132–40.
14. Petersenn S, Bollerslev J, Arafat AM, et al. Pharmacokinetics, pharmacody-namics and safety of pasireotide LAR in patients with acromegaly: a randomized, multicentre, open-label, Phase I study. J Clin Pharmacol 2014;54:1308–17.
15. Colao A, Bronstein MD, Freda P, et al. Pasireotide versus octreotide in acromegaly: a head-to-head superiority study. J Clin Endocrinol Metab 2014;99(3):791–9.
16. Gadelha M, Bronstein MD, Brue T, et al. Pasireotide versus continued treatment with octreotide or lanreotide in patients with inadequately controlled acromegaly (PAOLA): a randomized, phase 3 trial. Lancet Diabetes Endocrinol. 2014.
17. Flogstad AK, Halse J, Haldorsen T, et al. Sandostatin LAR in acromegalic patients: a dose-range study. J Clin Endocrinol Metab 1995;80(12):3601–7.
18. Shen G, Darstein D, Hermosillo Reséndiz K, et al. Pharmacokinetic and pharmaco-dynamic analyses of pasireotide LAR and octreotide LAR: randomized, double-blind, phase III study in patients with medically naïve acromegaly. 2014. Poster P918, Presented at the European Congress of Endocrinology, Wroclaw, Poland.
19. Schmid H, Brue T, Colao AM, et al, editor. Exploratory data evaluating the effect of pasireotide on GH, IGF-1, IGFBP-2, IGFBP-3, HbA1c and glucose in patients with inadequately controlled acromegaly enrolled in a 24-week study (PAOLA). ENDO meeting 2014. Chicago, June 21–24, 2014.

UPDATE 1: LATE-NIGHT SALIVARY CORTISOL IN DIAGNOSIS (SCREENING) OF ENDOGENOUS CUSHING SYNDROME

Endogenous Cushing syndrome is not common, but features of its phenotype are common.[4,5] The screening tests most commonly used are LNSC, the overnight low-dose dexamethasone test, and a 24-hour urine-free cortisol (UFC).[5] **Table 1** shows 2 previous diagnostic guidelines and my proposal for a diagnostic scheme centered on using LNSC as the primary initial test.[6,7] Over the past 10 to 15 years, the use of LNSC has matured into a widely used screening test, with high sensitivity and specificity.

In most situations, the measurement of LNSC has the greatest diagnostic accuracy and ease of use of tests commonly used to screen for endogenous Cushing syndrome.[8–19] This approach works because the diurnal nadir of cortisol secretion is usually not achieved with even mild Cushing syndrome, and salivary cortisol is a good surrogate for serum-free cortisol. Obtaining an LNSC sample is simple and can be performed at home in a low-stress environment. Immunoassays and liquid chromatography-tandem mass spectrometry (LC-MS/MS) have both been validated for the measurement of salivary cortisol, and the advantages and disadvantages of each are outlined in **Box 1**.[9,12,14,20–22]

Another advantage of the measurement of LNSC is its ability to identify patients with very mild endogenous Cushing syndrome.[23,24] Furthermore, assessment of LNSC in multiple longitudinal samples is a feasible approach to identify patients with intermittent, cyclic Cushing syndrome.[25] Salivary cortisol is useful to monitor the response to medical therapy for Cushing syndrome.[12,26]

Urinary cortisol excretion is a reasonable reflection of endogenous secretion, particularly when the hypothalamic-pituitary-adrenal axis is activated.[13,15,16,18] However, it lacks sensitivity and specificity and is too variable to be effective as a first-line screening test.[13,15,16,27,28] Most reference laboratories perform this analysis by LC-MS/MS, which, because of improved analytical specificity for cortisol, should improved diagnostic performance. However, several interfering substances have been identified using LC-MS/MS for the measurement of UFC,[29,30] and there are theoretic advantages to detecting steroid metabolites using immunoassays. Schemes using shorter collection times with normalization to urinary creatinine have been proposed.[25,31]

Table 1
Guidelines and current proposal for diagnosis of Cushing syndrome

	Arnaldi et al,[6] 2003	Neiman et al,[7] 2008	Current Proposal[8]
Initial diagnostic tests	24-h UFC (3 collections) LDDST (either type) LNSC (test not fully evaluated)	24-h UFC ($\geq$2 tests) 1-mg oDST LNSC ($\geq$2 tests)	LNSC (2 tests)
Confirmatory diagnostic tests (if necessary)	MSC Cortisol diurnal rhythm 2-mg LDDST $\pm$CRH test	2-mg LDDST Exclude physiologic causes Consult an endocrinologist Dexamethasone-CRH test or MSC	Repeat LNSC (2 tests) Test for contamination of saliva Confirm with UFC $\pm$ oDST

Abbreviations: CRH, corticotropin-releasing hormone; LDDST, low-dose dexamethasone test; MSC, midnight serum cortisol; oDST, overnight dexamethasone test.
Data from Refs.[6–8]

Box 1
Advantages and disadvantages of immunoassay versus LC-MS/MS for salivary cortisol

Immunoassay:

Advantages:

Better diagnostic sensitivity (92%) and specificity (96%)[11]

Simplicity (routine enzyme-linked immunosorbent assay) and low cost

Small sample volume requirement (40–50 μL)

Availability (cleared by US Food and Drug Administration)

Disadvantages:

Cross-reactivity with endogenous steroid metabolites (eg, cortisone) and synthetic steroids[8,9]

LC-MS/MS

Advantages:

Analytical specificity (measures only cortisol, not metabolites or prednisone)

Salivary cortisone can be measured[34,52]

Disadvantages:

Costly instrumentation and technically challenging

Lower diagnostic sensitivity (75%–91%) and specificity (90%)[14,21]

The premise of the low-dose dexamethasone suppression test is that endogenous cortisol hypersecretion is not suppressed by the administration of a physiologic dose of a glucocorticoid.[3] Immunoassays are usually adequate to detect suppressed 08:00 AM serum cortisol.[32,33] However, many patients with pituitary corticotroph adenomas suppress serum cortisol to less than 2 μg/dL (50 nmol/L) with low doses of dexamethasone,[23,33] so results of this test have to be interpreted with caution.

Table 2 compares the diagnostic tests described earlier using stringent criteria (sensitivity at 100% specificity and specificity at 100% sensitivity). Because LNSC performs well in most situations and is easy to execute, I propose that it be used as the initial test by immunoassay in patients with a diurnal lifestyle (**Fig. 1**). **Fig. 1** has not been vetted by a group of experts as have the guidelines in **Table 1**. If LNSC results by immunoassay do not fit the clinical scenario, samples can be reflexed to LC-MS/MS if contamination of the saliva sample by topical hydrocortisone is suspected.[34]

Table 2
Diagnostic characteristics of biochemical screening tests at 100% sensitivity and 100% specificity

Diagnostic Characteristic	Low-Dose Dexamethasone Suppression Test	24-h UFC	LNSC
Sensitivity (%) at 100% specificity	54	71	93
Specificity (%) at 100% sensitivity	41	73	96

Adapted from Findling JW, Raff H. Screening and diagnosis of Cushing's syndrome. Endocrinol Metab Clin North Am 2005;34(2):394; with permission.

12. Carrozza C, Lapolla R, Gervasoni J, et al. Assessment of salivary free cortisol levels by liquid chromatography with tandem mass spectrometry (LC-MS/MS) in patients treated with mitotane. Hormones (Athens) 2012;11(3):344–9.

13. Doi SA, Clark J, Russell AW. Concordance of the late night salivary cortisol in patients with Cushing's syndrome and elevated urine-free cortisol. Endocrine 2013; 43(2):327–33.

14. Erickson D, Singh RJ, Sathananthan A, et al. Late-night salivary cortisol for diagnosis of Cushing's syndrome by liquid chromatography/tandem mass spectrometry assay. Clin Endocrinol (Oxf) 2012;76(4):467–72.

15. Elias P, Martinez E, Barone B, et al. Late-night salivary cortisol has a better performance than urinary free cortisol in the diagnosis of Cushing's syndrome. J Clin Endocrinol Metab 2014;99:2045–51.

16. Manetti L, Rossi G, Grasso L, et al. Usefulness of salivary cortisol in the diagnosis of hypercortisolism: comparison with serum and urinary cortisol. Eur J Endocrinol 2013;168(3):315–21.

17. Nunes ML, Vattaut S, Corcuff JB, et al. Late-night salivary cortisol for diagnosis of overt and subclinical Cushing's syndrome in hospitalized and ambulatory patients. J Clin Endocrinol Metab 2009;94(2):456–62.

18. Raff H, Raff JL, Findling JW. Late-night salivary cortisol as a screening test for Cushing's syndrome. J Clin Endocrinol Metab 1998;83(8):2681–6.

19. Raff H. Utility of salivary cortisol measurements in Cushing's syndrome and adrenal insufficiency. J Clin Endocrinol Metab 2009;94(10):3647–55.

20. Miller R, Plessow F, Rauh M, et al. Comparison of salivary cortisol as measured by different immunoassays and tandem mass spectrometry. Psychoneuroendocrinology 2013;38(1):50–7.

21. Zerikly RK, Amiri L, Faiman C, et al. Diagnostic characteristics of late-night salivary cortisol using liquid chromatography-tandem mass spectrometry. J Clin Endocrinol Metab 2010;95(10):4555–9.

22. Palmieri S, Morelli V, Polledri E, et al. The role of salivary cortisol measured by liquid chromatography-tandem mass spectrometry in the diagnosis of subclinical hypercortisolism. Eur J Endocrinol 2013;168(3):289–96.

23. Kidambi S, Raff H, Findling JW. Limitations of nocturnal salivary cortisol and urine free cortisol in the diagnosis of mild Cushing's syndrome. Eur J Endocrinol 2007; 157(6):725–31.

24. Di DG, Vicennati V, Rinaldi E, et al. Progressively increased patterns of subclinical cortisol hypersecretion in adrenal incidentalomas differently predict major metabolic and cardiovascular outcomes: a large cross-sectional study. Eur J Endocrinol 2012;166(4):669–77.

25. Graham UM, Hunter SJ, McDonnell M, et al. A comparison of the use of urinary cortisol to creatinine ratios and nocturnal salivary cortisol in the evaluation of cyclicity in patients with Cushing's syndrome. J Clin Endocrinol Metab 2013; 98(1):E72–6.

26. Trementino L, Cardinaletti M, Concettoni C, et al. Salivary cortisol is a useful tool to assess the early response to pasireotide in patients with Cushing's disease. Pituitary 2014. http://dx.doi.org/10.1007/s11102-014-0557-x.

27. Lin CL, Wu TJ, Machacek DA, et al. Urinary free cortisol and cortisone determined by high performance liquid chromatography in the diagnosis of Cushing's syndrome. J Clin Endocrinol Metab 1997;82(1):151–5.

28. Petersenn S, Newell-Price J, Findling JW, et al. High variability in baseline urinary free cortisol values in patients with Cushing's disease. Clin Endocrinol (Oxf) 2014; 80(2):261–9.

29. Findling JW, Pinkstaff SM, Shaker JL, et al. Pseudohypercortisoluria: spurious elevation of urinary cortisol due to carbamazepine. Endocrinologist 1998;8:51–4.
30. Meikle AW, Findling J, Kushnir MM, et al. Pseudo-Cushing syndrome caused by fenofibrate interference with urinary cortisol assayed by high-performance liquid chromatography. J Clin Endocrinol Metab 2003;88(8):3521–4.
31. Shiwa T, Oki K, Yamane K, et al. Significantly high level of late-night free cortisol to creatinine ratio in urine specimen in patients with subclinical Cushing's syndrome. Clin Endocrinol (Oxf) 2013;79(5):617–22.
32. Barrou Z, Guiban D, Maroufi A, et al. Overnight dexamethasone suppression test: comparison of plasma and salivary cortisol measurement for the screening of Cushing's syndrome. Eur J Endocrinol 1996;134(1):93–6.
33. Findling JW, Raff H, Aron DC. The low-dose dexamethasone suppression test: a reevaluation in patients with Cushing's syndrome. J Clin Endocrinol Metab 2004; 89(3):1222–6.
34. Raff H, Singh RJ. Measurement of late-night salivary cortisol and cortisone by LC-MS/MS to assess preanalytical sample contamination with topical hydrocortisone. Clin Chem 2012;58(5):947–8.
35. Findling JW, Kehoe ME, Shaker JL, et al. Routine inferior petrosal sinus sampling in the differential diagnosis of adrenocorticotropin (ACTH)-dependent Cushing's syndrome: early recognition of the occult ectopic ACTH syndrome. J Clin Endocrinol Metab 1991;73(2):408–13.
36. Oldfield EH, Doppman JL, Nieman LK, et al. Petrosal sinus sampling with and without corticotropin-releasing hormone for the differential diagnosis of Cushing's syndrome. N Engl J Med 1991;325(13):897–905.
37. Aron DC, Raff H, Findling JW. Effectiveness versus efficacy: the limited value in clinical practice of high dose dexamethasone suppression testing in the differential diagnosis of adrenocorticotropin-dependent Cushing's syndrome. J Clin Endocrinol Metab 1997;82(6):1780–5.
38. Blevins LS Jr, Clark RV, Owens DS. Thromboembolic complications after inferior petrosal sinus sampling in patients with Cushing's syndrome. Endocr Pract 1998; 4(6):365–7.
39. Gandhi CD, Meyer SA, Patel AB, et al. Neurologic complications of inferior petrosal sinus sampling. AJNR Am J Neuroradiol 2008;29(4):760–5.
40. Swearingen B, Katznelson L, Miller K, et al. Diagnostic errors after inferior petrosal sinus sampling. J Clin Endocrinol Metab 2004;89(8):3752–63.
41. Daousi C, Nixon T, Javadpour M, et al. Inferior petrosal sinus ACTH and prolactin responses to CRH in ACTH-dependent Cushing's syndrome: a single centre experience from the United Kingdom. Pituitary 2010;13(2):95–104.
42. Findling JW, Kehoe ME, Raff H. Identification of patients with Cushing's disease with negative pituitary adrenocorticotropin gradients during inferior petrosal sinus sampling: prolactin as an index of pituitary venous effluent. J Clin Endocrinol Metab 2004;89(12):6005–9.
43. Mulligan GB, Eray E, Faiman C, et al. Reduction of false-negative results in inferior petrosal sinus sampling with simultaneous prolactin and corticotropin measurement. Endocr Pract 2011;17(1):33–40.
44. Sharma ST, Raff H, Nieman LK. Prolactin as a marker of successful catheterization during IPSS in patients with ACTH-dependent Cushing's syndrome. J Clin Endocrinol Metab 2011;96(12):3687–94.
45. Alexandraki KI, Kaltsas GA, Isidori AM, et al. Long-term remission and recurrence rates in Cushing's disease: predictive factors in a single-centre study. Eur J Endocrinol 2013;168(4):639–48.

46. Atkinson AB, Kennedy A, Wiggam MI, et al. Long-term remission rates after pituitary surgery for Cushing's disease: the need for long-term surveillance. Clin Endocrinol (Oxf) 2005;63(5):549–59.
47. Hameed N, Yedinak CG, Brzana J, et al. Remission rate after transsphenoidal surgery in patients with pathologically confirmed Cushing's disease, the role of cortisol, ACTH assessment and immediate reoperation: a large single center experience. Pituitary 2013;16(4):452–8.
48. Invitti C, Pecori GF, de Martin M, et al. Diagnosis and management of Cushing's syndrome: results of an Italian multicentre study. Study Group of the Italian Society of Endocrinology on the pathophysiology of the hypothalamic-pituitary-adrenal axis. J Clin Endocrinol Metab 1999;84(2):440–8.
49. Carrasco CA, Coste J, Guignat L, et al. Midnight salivary cortisol determination for assessing the outcome of transsphenoidal surgery in Cushing's disease. J Clin Endocrinol Metab 2008;93(12):4728–34.
50. Barbot M, Albiger N, Koutroumpi S, et al. Predicting late recurrence in surgically treated patients with Cushing's disease. Clin Endocrinol (Oxf) 2013;79(3): 394–401.
51. Abdelmannan D, Chaiban J, Selman WR, et al. Recurrences of ACTH-secreting adenomas after pituitary adenomectomy can be accurately predicted by perioperative measurements of plasma ACTH levels. J Clin Endocrinol Metab 2013; 98(4):1458–65.
52. Perogamvros I, Keevil BG, Ray DW, et al. Salivary cortisone is a potential biomarker for serum free cortisol. J Clin Endocrinol Metab 2010;95(11):4951–8.

Medical Treatment of Cushing Disease
New Targets, New Hope

Maria Fleseriu, MD[a,b],*

KEYWORDS

- Cushing disease • Medical therapy • Pasireotide • Mifepristone • LCI699
- Combination therapies

KEY POINTS

- For most patients with Cushing disease, transsphenoidal surgery remains the first-line therapy of choice; however, many patients will not achieve remission or will experience tumor recurrence.
- Pasireotide may be an attractive option as an initial medical therapy for some patients. Hyperglycemia is frequent but rarely severe; intense monitoring and timely treatment are required.
- Mifepristone may be appropriate in patients with diabetes mellitus, whereas patients with severe hypertension and uncontrolled hypokalemia are not good candidates.
- Several adrenal steroidogenesis inhibitors continue to be used off-label, with varying results.
- The value of medical combination therapy is still under investigation, and new medical therapies are in development.

INTRODUCTION

Cushing disease (CD) is a condition of hypercortisolism caused by a corticotropin (adrenocorticotropic hormone [ACTH])-secreting pituitary adenoma. If untreated, CD is associated with significant morbidity and mortality[1–3]; however, some investigators have suggested that early and aggressive intervention can increase survival.[2,3]

Dr M. Fleseriu is an ad hoc scientific consultant/advisor for Genentech, Novartis, and Pfizer. Her work is supported by research grants given to Oregon Health & Science University from Ipsen, Prolor, Novartis, and Cortendo.

[a] Department of Medicine (Endocrinology), Oregon Health & Science University, Mail Code BTE 28, 3181 Southwest Sam Jackson Park Road, Portland, OR 97239, USA; [b] Department of Neurological Surgery, Oregon Health & Science University, Mail Code BTE 28, 3181 Southwest Sam Jackson Park Road, Portland, OR 97239, USA

* Northwest Pituitary Center, Oregon Health & Science University, Mail Code BTE 28, 3181 Southwest Sam Jackson Park Road, Portland, OR 97239.

E-mail address: fleseriu@ohsu.edu

Endocrinol Metab Clin N Am 44 (2015) 51–70
http://dx.doi.org/10.1016/j.ecl.2014.10.006
0889-8529/15/$ – see front matter © 2015 Elsevier Inc. All rights reserved.

Successful patient management requires individualized and multidisciplinary care involving endocrinologists, neurosurgeons, radiation oncologists, and general surgeons (**Box 1**).[1,4,5]

For most CD patients, transsphenoidal surgery remains the first-line therapy of choice.[6] Other treatment modalities include medication, radiation therapy, and bilateral adrenalectomy.[1,6–8]

This article focuses on the most recent medical therapeutic advances, in particular newly approved ACTH modulators, a glucocorticoid receptor blocker, and a novel adrenal steroidogenesis inhibitor; other drugs are also discussed (**Table 1**).[1,6,7,9–15]

PITUITARY TARGETED MEDICAL THERAPY

Medications that exert effects at the level of the pituitary represent an appealing option for CD treatment.[16–19]

Somatostatin receptor ligands (SRLs) and dopamine agonists (DAs) that target corticotroph adenomas, which predominantly express somatostatin receptor (Sstr) subtype 5 and DA2 receptors, currently represent the 2 main classes of centrally acting drugs used to treat CD.

Somatostatin Receptor Ligand: Pasireotide (SOM230; Signifor)

Pasireotide (Novartis Pharmaceuticals, Basel Switzerland) is a cyclic hexapeptide with a high affinity for Sstrs 1, 2, 3, and 5[19–22]; affinity for Sstr 5 is 40-fold higher than other first-generation SRLs.[22]

Pasireotide reduces ACTH secretion in cell culture models and in cultured human corticotroph tumor cells.[23] In phase II and III studies, pasireotide was found to be efficacious in treating CD, although some limitations and adverse effects were recognized.

In a phase II, proof-of-concept, open-label, single-arm, 15-day multicenter study, pasireotide decreased urine free cortisol (UFC) levels in 76% of CD patients with direct effects on ACTH release. Hyperglycemia occurred in 36% of patients, some with pretreatment glucose abnormalities. Steady-state plasma pasireotide concentrations were achieved within 5 days of treatment. Intriguingly, responders appeared to have higher pasireotide exposure than nonresponders (**Box 2**).[8,21]

In a long-term extension to this study, the reductions in mean UFC persisted in all patients who were still taking the study drug at 2 years, albeit with an inherent selection bias for patients who continued in extension.[20]

Box 1
Therapy options in clinical practice

- Transsphenoidal surgery is the treatment of choice for most patients with Cushing disease
- If surgery fails, or the disease recurs, there are several possible treatment alternatives:
  - Medical therapy
  - Repeat surgery
  - Radiation and medical therapy
  - Bilateral adrenalectomy
- Lifelong monitoring for possible recurrence is required

Table 1
Medical therapy for Cushing disease

Drugs That:

Modulate ACTH Release	Inhibit Adrenal Steroidogenesis	Are a Glucocorticoid Receptor Antagonist	Had a Previous Limited Response and/or Are Not Presently Available
Dopamine agonist Cabergoline	Ketoconazole	Mifepristone[c]	Bromocriptine
	COR-003[b]		Octreotide
Somatostatin receptor	LCI699[b]		Valproic acid
ligand	Metyrapone		Cyproheptadine
Pasireotide[a] (SOM230)	Mitotane		Ketanserin
Retinoic acid[b]	Etomidate		Ritanserin
EGFR tyrosine kinase			Trilostane
inhibitor			Aminoglutethimide
Gefitinib[b]			Rosiglitazone
Cyclin-dependent kinase			
inhibitor			
R-roscovitine[b]			
(CYC202)			

All other drugs are used off-label for Cushing syndrome.
[a] Approved for Cushing disease by the Food and Drug Administration (FDA).
[b] Investigational use, in clinical trials.
[c] FDA approved for hyperglycemia associated with Cushing syndrome.
Data from Refs.[1,6,7,9–15]

Box 2
Pasireotide in clinical practice

- Pasireotide is a somatostatin receptor ligand approved for treatment of Cushing disease after surgery failure or when surgery is not an option
- Pasireotide (Signifor) is available in doses of 300, 600, 900 μg
- Administered as a subcutaneous injection, twice daily
- Starting dose 600 μg; further evaluation of clinical and biochemical response is required
- If response is not optimal, increase dose to 900 μg and reevaluate
- Most responding patients will do so within 2 to 3 months
- Evaluate glucose abnormalities before starting treatment; if hemoglobin A_{1c} (HbA1c) is elevated, consider aggressive management before starting pasireotide
- Discuss with patient the signs and symptoms of adrenal insufficiency
- Check fasting glucose, HbA1c, and liver function, and perform electrocardiography, before and during treatment as indicated
- Begin treatment if glucose abnormalities are detected
- If there are clinical signs of adrenal insufficiency, hold therapy and/or start replacement glucocorticoids if needed
- Frequent adverse events are listed in **Table 2**
- If there is no response to pasireotide alone, consider possible combination drug therapy or switching to another therapy

In the largest phase III clinical trial to date, in which 2 groups CD patients were randomized to pasireotide 600 µg and 900 µg with a possible uptitration of dose at month 3,[12] median UFC declined by almost half at 6 months, −47.9% (600 µg) and −47.9% (900 µg). However, UFC normalization at 6 months without a dose increase at 3 months was much lower: 15% (600 µg) and 26% (900 µg). Interestingly the uptitration only slightly increased the response rate to 16% and 29%, respectively. Of note, the response rate in mild CD (diagnosed as UFC >1.5–2 times the upper limit of normal) was higher, up to 50% in the 900-µg group, making this group of patients with mild biochemical disease potentially ideal candidates to begin this treatment. It is also feasible to identify patients who do not respond early on, which is reassuring for a drug with limited biochemical normalization rates. Plasma cortisol, ACTH, and night salivary cortisol also declined throughout the study, but somewhat less in comparison with the UFC levels.[12] Escape has not been noted, but longer-term data are limited[12,20]; one patient had long-term UFC control without escape or serious adverse events during more than 7 years of treatment.[24]

In parallel with the biochemical improvement, patients also showed significant improvements in signs and symptoms of hypercortisolism. Blood pressure decreased (systolic by 6.1 mm Hg and diastolic by 3.7 mm Hg), triglycerides and low-density lipoprotein cholesterol also improved, and patients lost weight (average 6.7 kg). At months 6 and 12, regression of facial rubor, supraclavicular fat pads, and dorsal fat pads were observed in patients with available photographs. Although the results are somewhat limited by the absence of a placebo group, health-related quality of life also increased significantly in most patients. Some patients noticed clinical improvement even in the absence of UFC normalization; however, achieving a normal UFC is still recommended.[25]

As expected from drugs acting on a pituitary tumor[12] and from the experience with SRLs in treating acromegaly, tumor shrinkage was noted after 1 year of treatment: −9.1% and −43.8% in the 600-µg and 900-µg groups, respectively.[12] Of note, many patients did not have measurable baseline pituitary tumor on MRI, and measuring changes in microadenomas can be difficult. Prospective studies with preoperative pasireotide treatment aimed at decreasing tumor size[26] (theoretically improving surgical outcome in patients with macroadenomas) have yet to be attempted. Further details on studies with pasireotide are presented in **Table 2**.[8,12–15,17,20,21,27–29]

Pasireotide long-acting release (LAR) is currently being studied in a large randomized, double-blind, multicenter, phase III study to evaluate efficacy and safety in CD patients (http://clinicaltrials.gov/show/NCT01374906).

Cabergoline and other drugs acting at the pituitary are reviewed in **Table 2**.[8,12–15,17,20,21,27–29]

Adrenal Steroidogenesis Inhibitors

Adrenal blocking drugs suppress cortisol production via inhibition of multiple steroidogenic enzymes. All are currently used as an off-label treatment for Cushing syndrome (CS).[5,10,30–32] Ketoconazole and metyrapone are most frequently used; but there are no prospective studies of these agents in CD patients.[18] Chronic treatment can be limited by side effects such as hepatotoxicity (ketoconazole) and increased androgen and mineralocorticoid production (metyrapone). The US Food and Drug Administration and the European Medicines Agency simultaneously issued, in 2013, a ketoconazole black-box warning for hepatotoxicity. Further details regarding dosing and adverse events are presented in **Table 3**.[6,8,10,11,17,18,31,33]

LCl699, a new potent inhibitor of both aldosterone synthase and 11β-hydroxylase, is currently under investigation in a prospective proof-of-concept study in patients with CD.[10,34] All but 1 of 12 patients had normalized UFC at a median LCl699 dose (5–10 mg twice daily for 10 weeks), although some patients required higher doses. Mean systolic and diastolic blood pressure decreased from baseline by 10 and 6 mm Hg, respectively. LCl699 was generally well tolerated; the most frequently reported adverse events were fatigue, nausea, and headache. Mean 11-deoxycortisol, 11-deoxycorticosterone, and ACTH levels increased during treatment and declined after discontinuation. Four of 12 patients experienced study drug–related mild hypokalemia (minimum 3.1 mmol/L). A longer-term, 22-week, multicenter open-label study, which included an expansion cohort in addition to the initial group (n = 19), confirmed the good remission rates, 78.9% of patients achieving normal UFC at week 22.[34] It is interesting that after the initial titration period, no responder required a dose increase between weeks 10 and 22. The most common long-term adverse events were asthenia and nasopharyngitis, and hypokalemia was observed in half of the patients. Hypocortisolism-related adverse events were reported in 6 patients. Hyperandrogenism, expected as a consequence of the mechanism of action, was noted in 4 women.[34] Based on these promising results, LCl699 may play a future role in the treatment of CD, and a phase III clinical trial to confirm efficacy and tolerability is planned (clinicaltrials.gov).

Glucocorticoid Receptor Blocker

Mifepristone directly blocks the glucocorticoid receptor and the progesterone receptor (affinity for the glucocorticoid receptor is more than 10-fold that of cortisol). It takes approximately 2 weeks to clear mifepristone from the circulation after dosing cessation.[30,35] Mifepristone use for refractory Cushing (but rarely in CD) was initially described in case reports and series.[8,30,36] A large open-label, 24-week, multicenter trial (SEISMIC) studied 50 mifepristone-treated CS patients, 43 with CD.[7] There were 2 mifepristone-treated (300–1200 mg; mean 900 mg) patient groups with either diabetes or hypertension. Overall, 60% of the patients with glucose intolerance or diabetes (n = 29) were responders. Glucose tolerance improved over time at each of the evaluations from week 6 to week 24, and 7 of 12 patients requiring insulin treatment were able to reduce their doses by at least 50% per day.[7] An independent data review determined that global clinical response was improved in 87% of patients.[37] Post hoc analysis of clinical response confirmed that mifepristone had a progressive clinical benefit, with a higher proportion of responses at study end (6 months). Of interest, a gender-dependent mifepristone effect was indicated; there was a more rapid clinical benefit in men, although there was no significant gender difference at study end.[37]

Data on both ACTH and corticotroph tumor size from the SEISMIC study and its long-term extension have been recently analyzed.[38,39] ACTH elevation during chronic therapy required several weeks to become maximal, but did not appear to be progressive with continued treatment. One-third of patients experienced a 4-fold or greater elevation in ACTH, whereas 11.6% of patients had little to no increase. Of 36 patients with more than one postbaseline magnetic resonance image, 17 had visible tumors, including 7 macroadenomas. Tumor progression occurred in 4 patients. One patient had early progression (week 10) of a large, aggressive macroadenoma, and 3 patients (2 macroadenoma, 1 microadenoma) had gradual tumor enlargement on long-term follow-up (20–36 months). Tumor regression was confirmed in 2 patients, 1 with a macroadenoma (status post radiation) and 1 with a microadenoma.[38,39] Increases in ACTH and a history of radiation therapy were not predictive of tumor increase.

Table 2
Neuromodulators of ACTH secretion: summary of study design and results

Authors,[Ref.] Year	Study Design and Drug Dose	Efficacy and Benefit	Adverse Effects and Limitations
Pasireotide			
Boscaro et al,[21] 2009	Prospective phase II trial; 15 d; N = 39 Dose: 600 µg twice daily	Reduced urinary free UFC levels in 76% of patients Normalized UFC in 17% of patients	Adverse effects similar to those of other somatostatin analogs, except degree and severity of hyperglycemia and diabetes mellitus
Boscaro et al,[20] 2013	Prospective phase II extension trial; N = 19 Open-ended, single-arm, multicenter extension, primary end point at 6 mo Dose: 600 and 900 µg, subcutaneous, twice daily	At extension (month 6) 56% of patients lower UFC than at core baseline, and 22% had normalized UFC Observed reductions in serum cortisol, plasma ACTH, body weight, and diastolic blood pressure	Bradycardia, abnormal LFTs rare Hypocortisolism-related adverse events in 13 (8%) patients
Colao et al,[12] 2012	Prospective phase III trial; 6 mo and extension; N = 162 Dose groups: 600 and 900 µg, subcutaneous, twice daily	Median UFC change from baseline was −47.9%; UFC normalization in 20.4%; higher rate of UFC normalization with lower baseline UFC Early identification of nonresponders: >90% of patients uncontrolled at months 1 and 2 remained uncontrolled at month 6 Serum and salivary cortisol and plasma ACTH levels decreased Clinical signs and symptoms of Cushing disease diminished	Phase III; common adverse events were diarrhea (58%), nausea (52%), cholelithiasis (30%), headache (28%), and abdominal pain (24%) Hyperglycemia-related adverse events in 118 of 162 patients Despite declines in cortisol levels, blood glucose and HbA1c increased soon after treatment initiation and then stabilized; 48% of nondiabetic patients had a glycated hemoglobin >6.5% at study end; treatment with a glucose-lowering medication was initiated in 74 of 162 patients Mechanism of pasireotide-induced hyperglycemia in healthy volunteers is now known to be due to decreases in insulin secretion and incretin hormone responses, without alterations in insulin sensitivity

Cabergoline

In vitro		If D2 receptors present 100% had significant ACTH secretion inhibition	
Pivonello et al,[15] 2009	Prospective; N = 20; 12–24 mo; oral. Dose: 1.5–7 mg/wk, oral. All patients had prior surgery	Initial remission in up to 75%; variable responses; at 24 mo, 40% of patients had normal UFC	Nausea, dizziness, hypotension, possible cardiac valvulopathy at high doses; escape from effect on cortisol
Lila et al,[28] 2010	Prospective; N = 18, 5 and 12 mo. Dose:1–5 mg/wk. Partial response: decrease of UFC to <125% of the ULN	Overall, 5 of 18 patients (28%) responded in terms of LDSC or MNSC (or both) at a mean dose of 3.6 mg/wk	
Godbout et al,[27] 2010	Retrospective; short (3–6 mo) and long (12–60 mo; mean 37) term. Dose: mean 2.1 mg/wk, maximum 6 mg/wk. Complete response: normal UFC	Response / Patient (n) / Patient (%): Complete short term 11 36.6; Partial 4 13.3; Complete long term 9 30. 2 patients experienced escape phenomenon after 2 and 5 y of complete response; however, 1 transiently renormalized UFC after an increase in cabergoline dosage. Potential positive metabolic effects (blood pressure, improvement of glucose tolerance), independently of cortisol-lowering effect	

Retinoic Acid

Pecori-Giraldi et al,[14] 2012	Prospective; N = 7, 6–12 mo, multicenter. Dose: escalating 10–80 mg/d	5 (71.4%) patients with ≥50% decrease/ normalization of UFC after 6 mo. 3 (42.9%) patients with marked and prolonged decrease in UFC. Blood pressure, glycemia, and signs of hypercortisolism, eg, body weight and facial plethora, were ameliorated to a variable extent	Patients reported only mild adverse effects, eg, xerophthalmia and arthralgias

(continued on next page)

Table 2
(continued)

Authors,[Ref.] Year	Study Design and Drug Dose	Efficacy and Benefit	Adverse Effects and Limitations
Temozolomide (Temodar)			
Raverot et al,[29] 2012	Case reports; aggressive ACTH-secreting tumors or ACTH carcinoma Doses: standard regimen of 150–200 mg/m² day; 5 d of a 28 d cycle for 3–24 cycles	Response to a trial of 3 cycles of treatment seemed sufficient to identify responders and was more reliable than patient MGMT status	Relatively well tolerated Fatigue, agranulocytosis, thrombocytopenia
Dillard et al,[46] 2011		ACTH decrease does not always correlate with tumor shrinkage Tumor shrinkage can be rapid Treatment escape?	
Getinifib			
Fukuoka et al,[13] 2011	In vitro and animal studies	Found to attenuate pro-opiomelanocortin expression, inhibit corticotroph tumor cell proliferation, and induce apoptosis in surgically resected human and canine corticotroph cultured tumors Decreased tumor size and corticosterone levels, and reversed signs of hypercortisolemia, including elevated glucose levels and excess omental fat in mice	Not applicable

Abbreviations: ACTH, corticotropin (adrenocorticotropin hormone); HbA1c, hemoglobin A_{1c}; LDSC, low-dose dexamethasone suppression serum cortisol; LFTs, liver function tests; MGMT, O^6-methylguanine-DNA methyltransferase; MNSC, midnight serum cortisol; UFC, urinary free cortisol; ULN, upper limit of normal.
Data from Refs.[8,12–15,17,20,21,27–29]

Table 3
Dosing and adverse events for adrenal steroidogenesis inhibitors

Drug	Activity/Enzyme(s) Inhibited	Dose	Overall Efficacy[a]	Pros	Cons	
Ketoconazole	Cholesterol side-chain cleavage 11β-Hydroxylase 17-Hydroxylase	Start at 200 mg/d ↑ As tolerated up to 400–1200 mg/d	53%–88% Castinetti et al,[11] 2014; N = 200, retrospective, multicenter 49.3% of patients had normal UFC levels 25.6% had at least a 50% decrease, and 25.4% had unchanged UFC levels Median final dose of ketoconazole 600 mg/d 41 patients (20.5%) stopped treatment because of poor tolerance	Rapid action Could take weeks to see full effect	Side effects GI Male hypogonadism Gastric acidity required for absorption Many drug-drug interactions Abnormal LFTs (serious AEs rare) Mild (<5-fold) and major (>5-fold) ↑ in liver enzymes observed in 13.5% and 2.5% of patients, respectively	Additional Black-box warning of possible liver toxicity 2–3 times/d dosing May be preferred in women
Metyrapone	11β-Hydroxylase	250–1000 mg 4 times a day Oral	75%, in small studies	Rapid action Cortisol levels ↓ within 2 h of initiating treatment	Side effects GI Hirsutism Hypertension Hypokalemia "Escape"?	Additional 4 times/d dosing Been used in pregnancy, but not approved

(continued on next page)

Table 3
(continued)

Drug	Activity/Enzyme(s) Inhibited	Dose	Overall Efficacy[a]	Pros	Cons	Additional
Mitotane	11β-Hydroxylase 18-Hydroxylase 3α-Hydroxylase Hydroxysteroid dehydrogenase Several cholesterol side-chain cleavage enzymes	0.5–3.0 g 3 times a day Oral Maximum dose in CD 1000 g 3 times a day	~70% Baudry et al,[31] 2012; retrospective, multicenter, N = 76 Remission was achieved in 48 (72%) of the 67 long-term treated patients, after a median time of 6.7 (5.2–8.2) mo 17 of 24 (71%) patients experienced recurrence, after a median time of 13.2 (5.0–67.9) mo A negative linear relationship was observed between plasma mitotane concentration and 24-h UFC (P<.0001)	Beneficial in adrenal cancer Also used in CD A pituitary adenoma became identifiable during mitotane treatment in 12 (25%) of the 48 patients with initial negative pituitary imaging, allowing subsequent transsphenoidal surgery	Side effects GI Liver abnormal Neurologic Teratogenic Adrenolytic Gynecomastia, rash Delayed efficacy Intolerance leading to treatment discontinuation occurred in 29% of patients	Additional Avoid in women desiring pregnancy within 5 y Mitotane doses may need to be reduced after 3 mo owing to saturation of fat tissue and subsequent overspill Look for minimal efficacious dose and avoid drug levels >20 μg/mL
Etomidate	Cholesterol side-chain cleavage 11β-Hydroxylase 17-Hydroxylase	0.03 mg/kg intravenous bolus Followed by 0.1–0.3 mg/kg/h	Case reports Useful particularly in cases with significant biochemical disturbance, sepsis, and other serious complications such as severe psychosis	Only parenteral drug available	Intensive ICU monitoring	

| LCI699[b] | 11β-Hydroxylase Aldosterone synthase | Median dose 10–20 mg/d Oral | 78.9%–92% Bertagna et al,[10] 2014; prospective, multicenter, open-label; N = 12 LCI699 started at 4 mg/d; the dose was escalated every 14 d to 10, 20, 40, and 100 mg/d until UFC normalized Dose was maintained until treatment ended (day 70) 11 (92%) had normal UFC Mean systolic and diastolic blood pressure ↓ from baseline by 10.0 and 6.0 mm Hg, respectively | Oral Shorter plasma half-life, therefore can be dosed 2 times a day rather than 3–4 times a day Higher potency compared with metyrapone | Mean 11-deoxycortisol, 11-deoxycorticosterone, and ACTH levels increased during treatment and declined after discontinuation Generally well tolerated Most AEs mild or moderate Most common AEs Fatigue (7/12) Nausea (5/12) Headache (3/12) Hypokalemia (25%) Hyperandrogenism in women could be expected owing to mechanism of action |

(continued on next page)

Table 3
(continued)

Drug	Activity/Enzyme(s) Inhibited	Dose	Overall Efficacy[a]	Pros	Cons
COR-003[b]	2S,4R enantiomer of ketoconazole Purified from racemic ketoconazole Significantly lower IC_{50} for 11β-hydroxylase and 14α-demethylase	Ongoing study Dose titration phase: ~2–16 wk Maintenance phase: 6 mo of treatment at therapeutic dose Extended evaluation phase: 6 mo of continued treatment after the maintenance phase (6–12 mo)	Single-period, open-label, dose-titration study to assess efficacy, safety, tolerability, and PK of COR-003 in subjects with CS Primary end point: mean UFC concentration ≤ULN following 6 mo of maintenance phase therapy without a prior dose increase during that phase	Expected to be a more potent inhibitor of key enzymes in the cortisol synthesis pathway Less potent inhibitor of a metabolic enzyme, CYP7A	No results yet available

Abbreviations: ↑, increase; ↓, decrease; AEs, adverse events; CD, Cushing disease; CS, Cushing syndrome; GI, gastrointestinal; ICU, intensive care unit; LFTs, liver function tests; PK, pharmacokinetics; UFC, urine free cortisol; ULN, upper limit of normal.

[a] Overall efficacy = from largest and most recent study to date.

[b] LCI investigational use proof-of-concept and extension phase, and COR-003 investigational use study design available on clinicaltrials.gov; adrenal steroidogenesis inhibitors used off-label and studied retrospectively.

Data from Refs.[6,8,10,11,17,18,31,33,46]

Additional long-term data from a larger number of patients are needed to provide further specifics (**Box 3**).

Combination Therapy

Corticotroph adenomas simultaneously express Sstr5 and dopamine D2 receptors.[19] In combining pasireotide with cabergoline, 2 pathways to inhibit tumoral ACTH secretion are targeted, and should achieve at least an additive effect. Synergistic effects in the treatment of CD have not been proved, although in vitro data suggest that this might occur via heterodimerization of Sstr5 and D2 receptors.[40]

The addition of cabergoline to pasireotide treatment in CD patients resulted in a further decrease of UFC values.[41] A large prospective pasireotide-cabergoline study is currently under way.[42] Cabergoline and ketoconazole have also been used in combination.[43,44] Sequential therapy using pasireotide, cabergoline, and ketoconazole shows promise, but requires analysis of efficacy and safety.[4]

Box 3
Mifepristone in clinical practice

- Mifepristone is a glucocorticoid receptor and progesterone receptor antagonist
- Mifepristone (Korlym; Corcept Therapeutics, Menlo Park, CA, USA) is approved by the Food and Drug Administration for the treatment of hyperglycemia associated with Cushing syndrome[7]
- Doses: 300, 600, 900, and 1200 mg daily
- Oral administration

Before Beginning Treatment

- Evaluate for hypokalemia: replace potassium, and start spironolactone if needed[7,31]
- Concomitant medication for interactions
- Review menstrual status, advise watching for any vaginal bleeding
- Review with patients clinical signs of adrenal insufficiency
- Contraindicated in patients planning pregnancy

Treatment

- Start mifepristone at 300 mg daily with food
- Further titration as needed based on clinical efficacy/tolerability
- Maximum daily dose 1200 mg

Monitoring

- Recheck potassium in 1 to 2 weeks
- Discuss higher dexamethasone dose, usually needed to treat adrenal insufficiency (up to 2–4 mg every 6–12 hours)[30]
- Cortisol is not a marker of efficacy and will be elevated; no need to monitor
- Vaginal ultrasonography may be necessary in women with vaginal bleeding
- Serial MRI as necessary, particularly in macroadenomas[28]
- Other adverse events include headache, nausea, reduction in high-density lipoprotein, and asymptomatic elevation of thyroid-stimulating hormone

After Discontinuation

- Antidiabetic, antihypertensive, and potassium doses may need to be adjusted

Table 4
Combination therapy studies for the treatment of Cushing disease

Authors,[Ref.] Year	Study Design	Study Drug Treatments					UFC and Salivary Cortisol Normalization	Clinical Improvements/ Study Comments	Select Adverse Events		
		SRLs	Cabergoline	Ketoconazole	Metyrapone	Mitotane			Hyperglycemia	Liver, GI Tract	Cardiac
Feelders et al,[41] 2010	N = 17 Prospective open-label stepwise multicenter Duration: up to 80 d Objective: normal UFC	Pasireotide 100–250 μg subcutaneous twice daily	Start 0.5 mg up to 1.5 mg oral every other day	200 mg thrice daily oral	X	X	88% and NA	↓ in body weight (−2.4 ± 0.9 kg), ↓ in waist circumference (−4.2 ± 1.3 cm), ↓ in systolic blood pressure (−12 ± 4 mm Hg), and ↓ in diastolic blood pressure (−8 ± 3 mm Hg)	HbA1c ↑ from 5.8 ± 0.2% to 6.7 ± 0.3%	NA	NA
Vilar et al,[44] 2010	N = 12 Prospective Duration: 9 mo	X	Max. dose: 3 mg/wk	200–400 mg/d oral	X	X	75% and NA	Regardless of UFC normalization, all patients reported	No	No	No

	Objective: biochemical control									
Kamenicky et al,[45] 2011	N = 11 Prospective open-label Inclusion based on severity Median follow-up 14 mo (range: 1–42) 4 subjects with CD Objective: efficacy and safety of combination therapy in severe ACTH-dependent CS	X	X	400–1200 mg/d oral divided doses Median dose 800 mg/24 h	3–4.5 g/d oral divided doses Median dose 3.0 g/24 h	3–5 g/d oral divided doses Median dose 3.0 g/24 h	UFC excretion ↓ rapidly from 2737 µg/24 h (range 853–22,605) at baseline to 50 µg/24 h (range 18–298) within 24–48 h Remained low to normal on combination and NA	Rapid and substantial improvement in the clinical features of CS Left ventricular function improved or normalized Oral hydrocortisone replacement therapy at a median dose of 32.5 mg/d (range 15–60)	GI; nausea and vomiting (63%) ↑ in γGT	DM 2 improved and/or doses of medications decreased	All patients initially had hypokalemia Lowest potassium concentration during treatment was 2.9 mmol/L (range 2.6–3.5) 9 patients required oral potassium supplementation and 8 required spironolactone ↑ in cholesterol
Van der Pas et al,[47] 2013	N = 17 Study design in Feelders et al,[41] 2010 Objective: cortisol rhythm and QoL	Pasireotide 100–250 µg Subcutaneous twice daily	Start 0.5 mg up to 1.5 mg oral every other day	200 mg oral thrice daily	X	X	NA and 50% recovery of diurnal rhythm	Baseline QoL was significantly impaired compared with literature-derived controls QoL did not improve or deteriorate after 80 d Cushing QoL scores seemed to improve	NA	HbA1c ↑ from 5.8 ± 0.2% to 6.7 ± 0.3%	NA

(continued on next page)

Table 4
(continued)

Authors,[Ref.] Year	Study Design	Study Drug Treatments					UFC and Salivary Cortisol Normalization	Clinical Improvements/ Study Comments	Select Adverse Events		
		SRLs	Cabergoline	Ketoconazole	Metyrapone	Mitotane			Liver, GI Tract	Hyperglycemia	Cardiac
								after 1 y of remission in 3 patients who continued medical therapy			
Barbot et al,[43] 2014	N = 14 Prospective 6 patients cabergoline then ketoconazole added 8 patients ketoconazole then cabergoline added Objective: combination	X	0.5–1 mg/wk up to 3.0 mg/wk	200 mg/d to 600 mg/d	X	X	79% and 28%	Partial regression in the signs of hypercortisolism, including reductions in waist circumference and BMI, decrease in number and/or dose of antihypertensive drugs	No	HbA1c ↓ from 0.3% to 3.2% after 6 mo of combined therapy	No

							Primary end point		
therapy effectiveness at relatively low doses and using different schedules									
Fleseriu,[42] 2014	N = 128 Prospective ongoing phase II multicenter international open-label noncomparative 2 treatment regimens (NCT01915303) Objective: effectiveness and safety of combination therapy in CD Changes in QoL, clinical signs and symptoms of CD	Pasireotide 300–600–900 µg twice daily	0.5–1 mg/d oral	X	X	X	Primary end point: proportion of responders (mean UFC ≤1.0 × ULN) Group 1 with pasireotide alone or with cabergoline at week 35 Group 2 with pasireotide in combination with cabergoline at week 17 Late night salivary cortisol to be determined	Clinical signs of hypercortisolism (facial rubor, supraclavicular and dorsal fat pads) to be evaluated using photographs Health-related QoL will be assessed using Cushing QoL and SF-12v2	NA	NA	NA

Abbreviations: ↑, increase; ↓, decrease; BMI, body mass index; CD, Cushing disease; CS, Cushing syndrome; DM 2, type 2 diabetes mellitus; HbA1c, hemoglobin A$_{1c}$; NA, not applicable; QoL, quality of life; SRLs, somatostatin receptor ligands; UFC, urine free cortisol; ULN, upper limit of normal.
Data from Refs.[41–45,47]

A combination of 3 adrenal steroidogenesis inhibitors (mitotane, metyrapone, and ketoconazole) as an alternative to urgent adrenalectomy has also been investigated.[45] The potential for combination of an agent that blocks adrenal steroidogenesis with inhibition of ACTH secretion by pasireotide needs further exploration (**Table 4**).[41–45]

SUMMARY

CD represents a significant challenge to physicians and patients alike. Newly approved medical therapy has changed the landscape; however, further research is required and progress needs to be made. Several compounds have the potential to significantly improve biochemical control and clinical phenotype. Combination drug therapy that targets different pathways seems to increase control rates with fewer adverse events. However, further ongoing research based on tumor receptor expression patterns is needed which, it is hoped, will lead to further improvements and new medical therapies specifically tailored to individual patients.

ACKNOWLEDGMENTS

The author thanks Andy Rekito, MS, and Shirley McCartney, PhD, for graphic and editorial assistance, respectively.

REFERENCES

1. Biller BM, Grossman AB, Stewart PM, et al. Treatment of adrenocorticotropin-dependent Cushing's syndrome: a consensus statement. J Clin Endocrinol Metab 2008;93:2454–62.
2. Clayton RN, Raskauskiene D, Reulen RC, et al. Mortality and morbidity in Cushing's disease over 50 years in Stoke-on-Trent, UK: audit and meta-analysis of literature. J Clin Endocrinol Metab 2011;96:632–42.
3. Feelders RA, Hofland LJ. Medical treatment of Cushing's disease. J Clin Endocrinol Metab 2013;98:425–38.
4. Trainer PJ. Next generation medical therapy for Cushing's syndrome-can we measure a benefit? J Clin Endocrinol Metab 2014;99:1157–60.
5. Fleseriu M, Loriaux DL, Ludlam WH. Second-line treatment for Cushing's disease when initial pituitary surgery is unsuccessful. Curr Opin Endocrinol Diabetes Obes 2007;14:323–8.
6. Nieman LK. Update in the medical therapy of Cushing's disease. Curr Opin Endocrinol Diabetes Obes 2013;20:330–4.
7. Fleseriu M, Biller BM, Findling JW, et al. Mifepristone, a glucocorticoid receptor antagonist, produces clinical and metabolic benefits in patients with Cushing's syndrome. J Clin Endocrinol Metab 2012;97:2039–49.
8. Tritos NA, Biller BM. Advances in medical therapies for Cushing's syndrome. Discov Med 2012;13:171–9.
9. Liu NA, Jiang H, Ben-Shlomo A, et al. Targeting zebrafish and murine pituitary corticotroph tumors with a cyclin-dependent kinase (CDK) inhibitor. Proc Natl Acad Sci U S A 2011;108:8414–9.
10. Bertagna X, Pivonello R, Fleseriu M, et al. LCI699, a potent 11beta-hydroxylase inhibitor, normalizes urinary cortisol in patients with Cushing's disease: results from a multicenter, proof-of-concept study. J Clin Endocrinol Metab 2014;99: 1375–83.
11. Castinetti F, Guignat L, Giraud P, et al. Ketoconazole in Cushing's disease: is it worth a try? J Clin Endocrinol Metab 2014. http://dx.doi.org/10.1210/jc.2013-3628.

12. Colao A, Petersenn S, Newell-Price J, et al. A 12-month phase 3 study of pasireotide in Cushing's disease. N Engl J Med 2012;366:914–24.
13. Fukuoka H, Cooper O, Ben-Shlomo A, et al. EGFR as a therapeutic target for human, canine, and mouse ACTH-secreting pituitary adenomas. J Clin Invest 2011;121:4712–21.
14. Pecori-Giraldi F, Ambrogio AG, Andrioli M, et al. Potential role for retinoic acid in patients with Cushing's disease. J Clin Endocrinol Metab 2012;97:3577–83.
15. Pivonello R, De Martino MC, Cappabianca P, et al. The medical treatment of Cushing's disease: effectiveness of chronic treatment with the dopamine agonist cabergoline in patients unsuccessfully treated by surgery. J Clin Endocrinol Metab 2009;94:223–30.
16. Fleseriu M, Petersenn S. New avenues in the medical treatment of Cushing's disease: corticotroph tumor targeted therapy. J Neurooncol 2013;114:1–11.
17. Fleseriu M, Petersenn S. Medical management of Cushing's disease: what is the future? Pituitary 2012;15:330–41.
18. Gadelha MR, Vieira Neto L. Efficacy of medical treatment in Cushing's disease: a systematic review. Clin Endocrinol (Oxf) 2014;80:1–12.
19. de Bruin C, Pereira AM, Feelders RA, et al. Coexpression of dopamine and somatostatin receptor subtypes in corticotroph adenomas. J Clin Endocrinol Metab 2009;94:1118–24.
20. Boscaro M, Bertherat J, Findling J, et al. Extended treatment of Cushing's disease with pasireotide: results from a 2-year, Phase II study. Pituitary 2013;17(4):320–6.
21. Boscaro M, Ludlam WH, Atkinson B, et al. Treatment of pituitary-dependent Cushing's disease with the multireceptor ligand somatostatin analog pasireotide (SOM230): a multicenter, phase II trial. J Clin Endocrinol Metab 2009;94:115–22.
22. Bruns C, Lewis I, Briner U, et al. SOM230: a novel somatostatin peptidomimetic with broad somatotropin release inhibiting factor (SRIF) receptor binding and a unique antisecretory profile. Eur J Endocrinol 2002;146:707–16.
23. Hofland LJ, van der Hoek J, Feelders R, et al. The multi-ligand somatostatin analogue SOM230 inhibits ACTH secretion by cultured human corticotroph adenomas via somatostatin receptor type 5. Eur J Endocrinol 2005;152:645–54.
24. Targher G. Pasireotide in Cushing's disease. N Engl J Med 2012;366:2134.
25. Pivonello R, Petersenn S, Newell-Price J, et al. Pasireotide treatment significantly improves clinical signs and symptoms in patients with Cushing's disease: results from a Phase III study. Clin Endocrinol (Oxf) 2014;81(3):408–17.
26. Shimon I, Rot L, Inbar E. Pituitary-directed medical therapy with pasireotide for a corticotroph macroadenoma: pituitary volume reduction and literature review. Pituitary 2012;15:608–13.
27. Godbout A, Manavela M, Danilowicz K, et al. Cabergoline monotherapy in the long-term treatment of Cushing's disease. Eur J Endocrinol 2010;163:709–16.
28. Lila AR, Gopal RA, Acharya SV, et al. Efficacy of cabergoline in uncured (persistent or recurrent) Cushing disease after pituitary surgical treatment with or without radiotherapy. Endocr Pract 2010;16:968–76.
29. Raverot G, Castinetti F, Jouanneau E, et al. Pituitary carcinomas and aggressive pituitary tumours: merits and pitfalls of temozolomide treatment. Clin Endocrinol (Oxf) 2012;76:769–75.
30. Fleseriu M, Molitch ME, Gross C, et al. A new therapeutic approach in the medical treatment of Cushing's syndrome: glucocorticoid receptor blockade with mifepristone. Endocr Pract 2013;19:313–26.

31. Baudry C, Coste J, Bou Khalil R, et al. Efficiency and tolerance of mitotane in Cushing's disease in 76 patients from a single center. Eur J Endocrinol 2012; 167:473–81.
32. Heyn J, Geiger C, Hinske CL, et al. Medical suppression of hypercortisolemia in Cushing's syndrome with particular consideration of etomidate. Pituitary 2012;15: 117–25.
33. Preda VA, Sen J, Karavitaki N, et al. Etomidate in the management of hypercortisolaemia in Cushing's syndrome: a review. Eur J Endocrinol 2012;167:137–43.
34. Pivonello R, Fleseriu M. Oral Presentation: LCI699, a potent 11β-hydroxylase inhibitor, normalizes urinary free cortisol levels in patients with Cushing's disease: 22-week, multicenter, open-label study. Chicago: ENDO; 2014.
35. Heikinheimo O, Kontula K, Croxatto H, et al. Plasma concentrations and receptor binding of RU 486 and its metabolites in humans. J Steroid Biochem 1987;26: 279–84.
36. Carmichael JD, Fleseriu M. Mifepristone: is there a place in the treatment of Cushing's disease? Endocrine 2013;44:20–32.
37. Katznelson L, Loriaux DL, Feldman D, et al. Global clinical response in Cushing's syndrome patients treated with mifepristone. Clin Endocrinol (Oxf) 2014;80: 562–9.
38. Fleseriu M, Findling JW, Koch CA, et al. Changes in plasma ACTH levels and corticotroph tumor size in patients with Cushing's disease during long-term treatment with the glucocorticoid receptor antagonist mifepristone. J Clin Endocrinol Metab 2014;99:3718–27.
39. Fleseriu M, Findling JW, Koch CA, et al. OR42-3 Changes in corticotroph tumor size and plasma ACTH levels in Cushing's disease (CD) patients during long-term treatment with the glucocorticoid antagonist mifepristone (MIFE). San Francisco (CA): The Endocrine Society; 2013.
40. Rocheville M, Lange DC, Kumar U, et al. Receptors for dopamine and somatostatin: formation of hetero-oligomers with enhanced functional activity. Science 2000;288:154–7.
41. Feelders RA, de Bruin C, Pereira AM, et al. Pasireotide alone or with cabergoline and ketoconazole in Cushing's disease. N Engl J Med 2010;362:1846–8.
42. Fleseriu M, Pivonello R, Pedroncelli AM, et al. Study Design of a Phase II Trial of Subcutaneous Pasireotide Alone or Combined with Cabergoline in Patients with Cushing's Disease, in Endocrine Society's 96th Annual Meeting and Expo. Chicago, 2014, MON-715.
43. Barbot M, Albiger N, Ceccato F, et al. Combination therapy for Cushing's disease: effectiveness of two schedules of treatment. Should we start with cabergoline or ketoconazole? Pituitary 2014;17:109–17.
44. Vilar L, Naves LA, Azevedo MF, et al. Effectiveness of cabergoline in monotherapy and combined with ketoconazole in the management of Cushing's disease. Pituitary 2010;13:123–9.
45. Kamenicky P, Droumaguet C, Salenave S, et al. Mitotane, metyrapone, and ketoconazole combination therapy as an alternative to rescue adrenalectomy for severe ACTH-dependent Cushing's syndrome. J Clin Endocrinol Metab 2011;96:2796–804.
46. Dillard TH, Gultekin SH, Delashaw JB Jr, et al. Temozolomide for corticotroph pituitary adenomas refractory to standard therapy. Pituitary 2011;14(1):80–91.
47. van der Pas R, de Bruin C, Pereira AM, et al. Cortisol diurnal rhythm and quality of life after successful medical treatment of Cushing's disease. Pituitary 2013;16(4): 536–44.

Prolactinomas

Andrea Glezer, MD, PhD, Marcello D. Bronstein, MD, PhD*

KEYWORDS

- Hyperprolactinemia • Prolactinoma • Pituitary tumors
- Hypogonadotropic hypogonadism • Infertility • Prolactin • Dopaminergic agonists

KEY POINTS

- Hyperprolactinemia is an important cause of infertility.
- Prolactinomas are the main pathologic cause of hyperprolactinemia.
- Medical treatment with dopamine agonists is effective and safe in most cases.
- Many current and potential future treatments may overcome the burden of aggressive and resistant prolactin-secreting tumors.

INTRODUCTION

Hyperprolactinemia is an important cause of galactorrhea, irregular menses, and infertility, especially among young women. The prolactin (PRL)-secreting pituitary adenoma (prolactinoma) is the most common pathologic cause of hyperprolactinemia. In patients harboring macroprolactinomas, besides hypogonadism-related symptoms, mass effect symptoms, such as other pituitary deficiencies and headache and visual disturbances, can also be found.

Besides prolactinomas, physiologic (pregnancy and lactation), pharmacologic (especially antipsychotics), systemic diseases (renal and hepatic failure), endocrine diseases (hypothyroidism, Cushing disease), other pituitary or sellar region tumors causing pituitary stalk disconnection, and macroprolactinemia can be the cause of hyperprolactinemia. More recently, PRL receptor mutation was described as a cause of hyperprolactinemia. Idiopathic hyperprolactinemia is diagnosed after ruling out all referred causes.

The identification of the correct cause of hyperprolactinemia is crucial for treatment. For example, in pharmacologic hyperprolactinemia, this can be achieved by discontinuing or switching the suspected drug. Concerning prolactinomas, dopamine agonist (DA) is the specific treatment of choice in most cases.

The authors have nothing to disclose.
Neuroendocrine Unit, Laboratory of Cellular and Molecular Endocrinology LIM-25, Division of Endocrinology and Metabolism, Hospital das Clinicas, University of São Paulo Medical School, Rua Enéas de Carvalho Aguiar, São Paulo CEP 05403-000, Brazil
* Corresponding author. Rua Enéas de Carvalho Aguiar, 155 8 Andar Bloco 03, São Paulo CEP 05403-000, Brazil.
E-mail address: mdbronstein@uol.com.br

EPIDEMIOLOGY

Prolactinoma is the most common pituitary tumor. Its estimated prevalence is 500 cases per million and incidence of 27 cases per million per year. Microadenomas correspond to 60% of the cases prevailing in women. Adolescents and men usually harbor macroadenomas. PRL-secreting carcinomas are extremely rare.[1]

PATHOPHYSIOLOGY

PRL is under dopaminergic inhibitory tonus coming from tuberoinfundibular-pituitary neurons. Dopamine acts through dopamine receptor type 2, especially the short isoform, reducing PRL transcription and secretion, and reducing lactotroph proliferation.[2] However, various factors stimulate PRL secretion by inhibiting dopamine tonus, such as opioids, cholecystokinin, bombesin, neurotensin, and neuropeptide Y; or by directly stimulating PRL secretion, such as vasoactive intestinal peptide, breastfeeding, and stress.[3] Estrogens stimulate PRL secretion acting directly in the lactotrophs and also reducing dopaminergic activity by increasing expression of the less active long isoform of the D_2 receptor.[2] Hyperprolactinemia causes hypogonadism mainly by inhibiting pulsatile gonadotropin-releasing hormone secretion, in addition to direct inhibition of gonadal steroidogenesis.[4] It was recently demonstrated in rodents that PRL directly acts on hypothalamic neurons by inhibiting the expression of the gene Kiss1 kisspeptin, and this could be the possible mechanism responsible for reducing secretion of gonadotropin-releasing hormone.[5] Signs and symptoms related to hyperprolactinemia are present in physiologic states, such as pregnancy and breastfeeding, and in pharmacologic and pathologic cases.

CLINICAL FEATURES

Signs and symptoms found in patients with hyperprolactinemia are related to hypogonadotropic hypogonadism and galactorrhea. Galactorrhea is not a specific signal and may be present in individuals with normal PRL levels.[6] Hypogonadism can cause menstrual irregularity and amenorrhea in women, sexual dysfunction, infertility, and loss of bone mineral mass in both genders. Hyperprolactinemia is an important cause of infertility in clinical practice. In women, it can be characterized by short luteal phase, anovulatory cycles, oligomenorrhea, and amenorrhea, whereas in men, changes in viability and quantity of sperm can occur.[7] Hyperprolactinemia can also reduce libido independently of testosterone levels.[8,9] Patients with hyperprolactinemia often have reduced bone mineral density,[10] which may lead to fractures in both sexes. In patients with macroprolactinomas, besides the implications related to hormonal hypersecretion, tumor mass effect symptoms, such as headache, visual changes, and hydrocephalus, can also occur. Hypopituitarism beyond hypogonadism can occur if there is compression of the pituitary stalk or destruction of normal pituitary tissue.[11,12]

DIAGNOSIS

In patients with signs and symptoms related to hyperprolactinemia, evaluation of serum PRL is required. Usually, in prolactinomas, PRL level is proportional to the tumor mass: 50 to 300 ng/mL in microprolactinomas and 200 to 5000 ng/mL in macroprolactinomas (normal range, 2–23 ng/mL). However, disproportion between PRL levels and tumor mass can be found in cystic prolactinomas and giant prolactinomas because of "hook effect" (discussed later). Provocative tests, such as thyrotropin-releasing hormone and metoclopramide, or even suppression test with L-dopa are no longer used in clinical practice because they do not help the differential diagnosis.[13] In pituitary tumors, except for prolactinomas, and in other tumors of the sellar region, pituitary stalk disconnection may occur with consequent loss of the inhibitory effect of dopamine in the lactotrophs, resulting in hyperprolactinemia. Nevertheless, PRL levels in those situations rarely exceed 100 ng/mL.[14,15] The differential diagnosis between prolactinomas and the so-called "pseudoprolactinomas" is critical to point to the correct treatment, medical for prolactinomas and surgical for other tumors and the clinically nonfunctioning ones.

Giant prolactinomas in general present with extremely high PRL levels, greater than 4000 ng/mL, which can cause a laboratorial artifact in PRL serum measurement by immunometric assays underestimating the real value, known as "hook effect." Serum dilution can prevent this diagnostic pitfall.[16,17]

Another cause of clinical and laboratory dissociation is macroprolactinemia. PRL isoforms can be classified according to their molecular weight as monomeric, dimeric, and macroprolactin (big-bigPRL). Typically, the most prevalent isoform is monomeric, followed by dimeric, being macroprolactin less than 5% of total PRL. However, in 10% and 25% of patients with hyperprolactinemia, the major circulating isoform is macroprolactin, a situation known as macroprolactinemia.[18] Macroprolactin, mostly formed by a complex of IgG bound to PRL, has low biologic activity,[19] being macroprolactinemia, a benign condition. However, macroprolactinemia can coexist with elevated serum levels of monomeric PRL, leading to symptomatic hyperprolactinemia.[20] In this situation, additional imaging and laboratory research are required. The screening of macroprolactinemia is routinely performed by dosing serum PRL recovery after treatment with polyethylene glycol.

In a patient with hyperprolactinemia, after excluding pregnancy, breastfeeding, pharmacologic causes, primary hypothyroidism, and renal and hepatic impairment, it is recommended to perform an MRI,[13] which may detect a microprolactinoma (<1 cm) or a macroprolactinoma (>1 cm). Giant prolactinomas are defined when the maximal diameter is greater than 4 cm. If a macroprolactinoma causes optic chiasmal compression, a neuro-ophthalmologic evaluation is indicated. Because hyperprolactinemia can cause hypogonadism and reduced bone mineral density, bone densitometry should be performed and repeated, if necessary.

Additional pituitary function should be assessed, especially in macroprolactinomas, including insulinlike growth factor 1 measurements to evaluate the possibility of tumoral growth hormone (GH) cosecretion. Serum gonadotropin levels may be normal or suppressed, reflecting hypogonadotropic hypogonadism. In patients with prolactinomas, screening for multiple endocrine neoplasia type 1 is also recommended.[21] Because the issue of valvular heart disease associated with the use of DAs for prolactinomas is still an open question, we recommend performing a transthoracic echocardiogram before the initiation and periodically depending on the dose and duration of treatment.

TREATMENT

Goals of prolactinoma treatment include normalization of serum PRL levels and reduction of tumor size in macroprolactinomas, aiming at eugonadism restoration and reversion of mass effects that lead to headache, visual disturbances, and hypopituitarism. Treatment modalities are DA, neurosurgery, and radiotherapy.

DAs are the gold standard treatment of prolactinoma, because its use controls hormonal secretion and tumor growth in about 80% of cases. Cabergoline (CAB), a specific agonist of the D_2 receptor, is the first choice because of its greater efficacy and better tolerability. Bromocriptine use leads to normal serum PRL levels in 80% of microprolactinomas and 70% of macroprolactinomas, whereas with CAB this objective is achieved in 85% of patients.[22] The most common side effects are nausea, vomiting, and postural hypotension. Rarely nasal congestion, cramps, and psychiatric disorders may develop. CAB, in much higher doses than those commonly used in hyperprolactinemia, was related to valvulopathy in patients with Parkinson disease. Because CAB is also an agonist of the serotonin receptor 5HT2B it can promote valvar fibroblasts proliferation and, consequently, valvular insufficiency, especially in tricuspid and pulmonary valves. In patients using CAB for the treatment of hyperprolactinemia, the association with valvular heart disease is still controversial. In a recent review,[23] no risk of valve failure associated with the use of CAB was observed in most studies. Nevertheless, a greater risk of mild to moderate regurgitation usually in tricuspid valve has been reported in some publications, one study reporting moderate risk of dose-dependent tricuspid regurgitation.[24] In recent studies, bromocriptine has also been implicated with subclinical valvular fibrosis, and therefore may not be a safe alternative for patients on CAB with newly diagnosed or preexisting valvular relevant abnormalities.[25,26] Quinagolide, a nonergot DA only available in Europe, could be an alternative, but no data on this issue are published to date. Although a matter of controversy, we suggest this procedure before and periodically during use of DA, at the physician's discretion.

Remission of hyperprolactinemia may occur after DA treatment. In a recent meta-analysis, Dekkers and colleagues[27] showed that on average, 21% of patients with microprolactinomas or macroprolactinomas treated with DA maintained normoprolactinemia after drug discontinuation. Therefore, in patients presenting with normorprolactinemia and tumor reduction, it is worth trying to withdraw the drug, especially after 2 years of treatment.[13]

Surgical Treatment

Surgery, usually by the transsphenoidal approach, is indicated for patients with resistance or intolerance to DA; macroprolactinomas with chiasmal compression and visual impairment without fast improvement by medical treatment; symptomatic apoplexy; cerebrospinal fluid leak, which can occur in cases of invasion of the sphenoid sinus; and tumor shrinkage with the use of DA. In a recent review, more than 90% of cases of cerebrospinal fluid leakage were related to the use of DA, with a mean time of 3.3 months between the start of drug administration and the diagnosis of rhinorrhea,[28] although it was already reported that this treatment complication can occur during long-term treatment.[29] The experience of the neurosurgeon, moderately increased serum PRL levels (<200 ng/mL), and tumor size and invasiveness are the most important determinants of successful surgical treatment. In a literature review, prolactinoma remission occurred on average in 74.7% and 34% in microprolactinomas and macroprolactinomas, with a recurrence rate of 18% and 23%, respectively.[30] Tumor debulking is a strategy that has been successfully used for other pituitary adenomas, such as somatotropinomas.[31] In two recent studies, the authors showed that many patients with partial resistance to CAB achieve PRL normalization after surgical debulking, using a lower dose of CAB.[32,33]

Radiotherapy

Prolactinomas are among the most radioresistant pituitary tumors. Therefore, radiation therapy is only indicated to control tumor growth in DA-resistant cases not controlled by surgery. PRL normalization occurs in 31.4% of cases, and there was no difference in efficacy between conventional and stereotactic techniques.[30,34] Side effects include hypopituitarism, optic nerve injury, neuropsychiatric disorders, cerebrovascular disease, and development of secondary tumors.

Management of Aggressive Prolactinoma

Aggressive prolactinomas are characterized by the presence of expansion or invasion of neighboring structures, rapid tumor growth, and/or the presence of a tumor more than 4 cm in diameter. Many of them are resistant to DA. The first strategy to treat patients partially resistant to DA is a gradual increase in the dose of medication. Although the use of more than 2 mg per week of CAB is off label, Ono and colleagues[35] achieved normalization of PRL levels in 96.2% of patients with doses up to 12 mg per week of CAB.[13] Another strategy is the use of temozolomide, an oral alkylating agent that crosses the blood-brain barrier. In a recent review of the literature[36] there was response in 15 of 20 cases of PRL-secreting pituitary adenomas or carcinomas on temozolomide. The response was correlated to the absence of the methylguanine methyltransferase studied by immunohistochemistry. The methylguanine methyltransferase is a DNA repair enzyme that neutralizes the effect of temozolomide chemotherapy, but the influence of this presence as a prognosis factor is still controversial. Other treatment strategies undergoing clinical trials are the use of chimeric molecules (somatostatin analogues and dopamine D_2 receptors); multiligant somatostatin analogs, such as pasireotide[37]; estrogen receptor modulators[38]; PRL receptor antagonists[39]; and antiblastic drugs, such as mTOR and tyrosine kinase inhibitors.[40]

Prolactinomas, Fertility, and Pregnancy

Fertility is restored in most women with the use of DA. Nevertheless, in the absence of hormonal control in cases with microprolactinomas, clomiphene citrate or recombinant gonadotropins may be used for ovulation induction.[41] During pregnancy, the primary concern is growth of the tumor, because of high levels of estrogens, leading to visual disturbance and headache. In microprolactinomas, the chance of clinically significant tumor growth is less than 5%, and therefore, after pregnancy confirmation, DA can be withdrawn and the patient should be monitored clinically every trimester. In the presence of headache or visual changes, sellar MRI without gadolinium enhancement should be performed, preferentially after the first trimester of pregnancy. If there is a significant tumor growth, DA should be reintroduced. However, in patients with macroadenomas, the risk of tumor growth with clinical repercussion is up to 35%. Thus, in patients with expansive macroprolactinomas, it is mandatory to observe a tumor within the sellar boundaries, and usually to wait at least 1 year with treatment with DA. When tumor reduction does not occur, surgical treatment is indicated before allowing pregnancy.

The maintenance or not of DA during pregnancy should be a decision of the specialist. Neuro-ophthalmologic assessment should be performed periodically. In a case with tumor growth after DA withdrawal, the initial procedure is the reintroduction of the drug. In case of failure, surgical treatment is indicated, preferably in the second trimester.[42]

In men, in addition to sexual dysfunction, hyperprolactinemia can cause changes in sperm quality, especially in relation to motility. A period of CAB treatment beyond that required for achieving normal levels of testosterone is usually necessary for improving sperm quality.[43] In patients who remain with hypogonadism, clomiphene citrate has proved useful in increasing testosterone levels, even in the absence of normal serum

PRL levels. This approach has advantages over testosterone replacement regarding fertility restoration.[44]

MANAGEMENT

In a patient with signs and symptoms related to hyperprolactinemia, serum PRL levels must be performed and after hyperprolactinemia confirmation, clinical and laboratorial work-up to identify possible causes is necessary. After ruling out pregnancy, lactation, drug-related hyperprolactinemia, renal or hepatic insufficiency, and hypothyroidism, a sellar MRI is indicated. In general, in patients with microprolactinomas and especially macroprolactinomas, DA use could be introduced gradually. Except when pregnancy is desired, CAB is the preferential choice.[45] The dose can be titrated slowly, according to serum PRL levels monthly to every three months, from 0.25 mg once or twice a week to 2 mg a week. If there is visual deficiency, a new evaluation can be performed in days or weeks. Sellar MRI should be repeated depending on tumor characteristics at the physician's discretion.

REFERENCES

1. Bronstein MD. Disorders of prolactin secretion and prolactinomas. In: DeGroot LJ, Jameson JL, editors. Endocrinology. 6th edition. Philadelphia: Saunders/Elsevier; 2010. p. 333–57.
2. Ben-Jonathan N, Hnasko R. Dopamine as a prolactin (PRL) inhibitor. Endocr Rev 2001;22(6):724–63.
3. Freeman ME, Kanyicska B, Lerant A, et al. Prolactin: structure, function, and regulation of secretion. Physiol Rev 2000;80(4):1523–631.
4. Vlahos NP, Bugg EM, Shamblott MJ, et al. Prolactin receptor gene expression and immunolocalization of the prolactin receptor in human luteinized granulose cells. Mol Hum Reprod 2001;7:1033–8.
5. Sonigo C, Bouilly J, Carré N, et al. Hyperprolactinemia-induced ovarian acyclicity is reversed by kisspeptin administration. J Clin Invest 2012;122(10):3791–5.
6. Marshall JC, Dalkin AC, Haisenleder DJ, et al. GnRH pulses: the regulators human reproduction. Trans Am Clin Climatol Assoc 1993;104:31–46.
7. Kleinberg DL, Noel GL, Frantz AG. Galactorrhea: a study of 235 cases, including 48 with pituitary tumors. N Engl J Med 1977;296(11):589–600.
8. Corona G, Mannucci E, Fisher AD, et al. Effect of hyperprolactinemia in male patients consulting for sexual dysfunction. J Sex Med 2007;4:1485–93.
9. Buvat J. Hyperprolactinemia and sexual function in men: a short review. Int J Impot Res 2003;15:373–7.
10. Koppelman MC, Kurtz DW, Morrish KA, et al. Vertebral body bone mineral content in hyperprolactinemia women. J Clin Endocrinol Metab 1984;59(6):1050–3.
11. Mah PM, Webster J. Hyperprolactinemia: etiology, diagnosis, and management. Semin Reprod Med 2002;20(4):365–74.
12. Poon A, McNeill P, Harper A, et al. Patterns of visual loss associated with pituitary macroadenomas. Aust N Z J Ophthalmol 1995;23(2):107–15.
13. Melmed S, Casanueva FF, Hoffman AR, et al, Endocrine Society. Diagnosis and treatment of hyperprolactinemia: an Endocrine Society clinical practice guideline. J Clin Endocrinol Metab 2011;96(2):273–88.
14. Karavitaki N, Thanabalasingham G, Shore HC, et al. Do the limits of serum prolactin in disconnection hyperprolactinaemia need re-definition? A study of 226 patients with histologically verified non-functioning pituitary macroadenoma. Clin Endocrinol (Oxf) 2006;65(4):524–9.

15. Behan LA, O'Sullivan EP, Glynn N, et al. Serum prolactin concentration at presentation of non-functioning pituitary macroadenomas. J Endocrinol Invest 2013; 36(7):50814.
16. Frieze TW, Mong DP, Koops MK. "Hook effect" in prolactinomas: case report and review of literature. Endocr Pract 2002;8(4):296–303.
17. St-Jean E, Blain F, Comtois R. High prolactin levels may be missed by immunoradiometric assay in patients with macroprolactinomas. Clin Endocrinol (Oxf) 1996;44(3):305–9.
18. Shimatsu A, Hattori N. Macroprolactinemia: diagnostic, clinical, and pathogenic significance. Clin Dev Immunol 2012;2012:167132.
19. Glezer A, Soares CR, Vieira JG, et al. Human macroprolactin displays low biological activity via its homologous receptor in a new sensitive bioassay. J Clin Endocrinol Metab 2006;91(3):1048–55.
20. Bronstein MD. Editorial: is macroprolactinemia just a diagnostic pitfall? Endocrine 2012;41(2):169–70.
21. Delemer B. MEN1 and pituitary adenomas. Ann Endocrinol (Paris) 2012;73(2): 59–61.
22. Webster J, Piscitelli G, Polli A, et al. A comparison of cabergoline and bromocriptine in the treatment of hyperprolactinemic amenorrhea. Cabergoline Comparative Study Group. N Engl J Med 1994;331:904–9.
23. Valassi E, Klibanski A, Biller BM. Potential cardiac valve effects of dopamine agonists in hyperprolactinemia. J Clin Endocrinol Metab 2010;95(3):1025–33.
24. Colao A, Galderisi M, Di Sarno A, et al. Increased prevalence of tricuspid regurgitation in patients with prolactinomas chronically treated with cabergoline. J Clin Endocrinol Metab 2008;93(10):3777–84.
25. Boguszewski CL, dos Santos CM, Sakamoto KS, et al. A comparison of cabergoline and bromocriptine on the risk of valvular heart disease in patients with prolactinomas. Pituitary 2012;15(1):44–9.
26. Elenkova A, Shabani R, Kalinov K, et al. Increased prevalence of subclinical cardiac valve fibrosis in patients with prolactinomas on long-term bromocriptine and cabergoline treatment. Eur J Endocrinol 2012;167(1):17–25.
27. Dekkers OM, Lagro J, Burman P, et al. Recurrence of hyperprolactinemia after withdrawal of dopamine agonists: systematic review and meta-analysis. J Clin Endocrinol Metab 2010;95(1):43–51.
28. Lam G, Mehta V, Zada G. Spontaneous and medically induced cerebrospinal fluid leakage in the setting of pituitary adenomas: review of the literature. Neurosurg Focus 2012;32(6):E2.
29. Bronstein MD, Musolino NR, Benabou S, et al. Cerebrospinal fluid rhinorrhea occurring in long-term bromocriptine treatment for macroprolactinomas. Surg Neurol 1989;32(5):346–9.
30. Gillam MP, Molitch ME, Lombardi G, et al. Advances in the treatment of prolactinomas. Endocr Rev 2006;27(5):485–534.
31. Jallad RS, Musolino NR, Kodaira S, et al. Does partial surgical tumour removal influence the response to octreotide-LAR in acromegalic patients previously resistant to the somatostatin analogue? Clin Endocrinol (Oxf) 2007;67(2):310–5.
32. Vroonen L, Jaffrain-Rea ML, Petrossians P, et al. Prolactinomas resistant to standard doses of cabergoline: a multicenter study of 92 patients. Eur J Endocrinol 2012;167(5):651–62.
33. Primeau V, Raftopoulos C, Maiter D. Outcomes of transsphenoidal surgery in prolactinomas: improvement of hormonal control in dopamine agonist-resistant patients. Eur J Endocrinol 2012;66(5):779–86.

34. Sheplan Olsen LJ, Robles Irizarry L, Chao ST, et al. Radiotherapy for prolactin-secreting pituitary tumors. Pituitary 2012;15(2):135–45.
35. Ono M, Miki N, Kawamata T, et al. Prospective study of high-dose cabergoline treatment of prolactinomas in 150 patients. J Clin Endocrinol Metab 2008; 93(12):4721–7.
36. Whitelaw BC, Dworakowska D, Thomas NW, et al. Temozolomide in the management of dopamine agonist-resistant prolactinomas. Clin Endocrinol (Oxf) 2012; 76(6):877–86.
37. Hofland LJ, van der Hoek J, van Koetsveld PM, et al. The novel somatostatin analog SOM230 is a potent inhibitor of hormone release by growth hormone- and prolactin-secreting pituitary adenomas in vitro. J Clin Endocrinol Metab 2004;89(4):1577–85.
38. Heaney AP, Fernando M, Melmed S. Functional role of estrogen in pituitary tumor pathogenesis. J Clin Invest 2002;109(2):277–83.
39. Goffin V, Touraine P, Culler MD, et al. Drug insight: prolactin-receptor antagonists, a novel approach to treatment of unresolved systemic and local hyperprolactinemia? Nat Clin Pract Endocrinol Metab 2006;2(10):571–81.
40. Fukuoka H, Cooper O, Mizutani J, et al. HER2/ErbB2 receptor signaling in rat and human prolactinoma cells: strategy for targeted prolactinoma therapy. Mol Endocrinol 2011;25(1):92–103.
41. Serafini P, Motta EL, White JS. Restoration of ovarian cyclicity and ovulation induction in hypopituitary women. In: Bronstein MD, editor. Pituitary tumors in pregnancy. Boston (MA): Kluwer Academic Publishers; 2001. p. 173–94.
42. Bronstein MD, Paraiba DB, Jallad RS. Management of pituitary tumors in pregnancy. Nat Rev Endocrinol 2011;7(5):301–10.
43. Colao A, Vitale G, Cappabianca P, et al. Outcome of cabergoline treatment in men with prolactinoma: effects of a 24-month treatment on prolactin levels, tumor mass, recovery of pituitary function, and semen analysis. J Clin Endocrinol Metab 2004;89(4):1704–11.
44. Ribeiro RS, Abucham J. Recovery of persistent hypogonadism by clomiphene in males with prolactinomas under dopamine agonist treatment. Eur J Endocrinol 2009;161(1):163–9.
45. Glezer A, Bronstein MD. Prolactinomas, cabergoline, and pregnancy. Endocrine 2014;47(1):64–9.

Silent Pituitary Adenomas

Sarah E. Mayson, MD[a], Peter J. Snyder, MD[b],*

KEYWORDS

- Nonfunctioning pituitary adenoma • Silent pituitary adenoma
- Clinically silent pituitary adenoma

KEY POINTS

- Nonfunctioning, or silent, pituitary adenomas can arise from any anterior pituitary cell type and may be "clinically silent" or "totally silent."
- Gonadotroph and null-cell adenomas are the most prevalent type of silent pituitary adenomas.
- Silent adenomas that are associated with neurologic defects require transsphenoidal surgery; radiation therapy may be used to treat residual or recurrent disease.

INTRODUCTION

Pituitary adenomas are uncommon. A cross-sectional study from the United Kingdom found that the prevalence of pituitary adenomas was 77.6 per 100,000 people.[1] They can arise from any anterior pituitary cell type. Some pituitary adenomas cause clinical manifestations related to the excessive secretion of their hormonal products, whereas others are nonfunctioning or "silent" (**Box 1**). Although they are common among pituitary adenomas, the annual incidence of nonfunctioning pituitary adenomas is only approximately 1.5 per 100,000 people.[2]

TYPES OF SILENT PITUITARY ADENOMAS

Pituitary adenomas are classified based on the anterior pituitary cell type of origin (**Table 1**).

- Adenomas can therefore be lactotroph, somatotroph, corticotroph, gonadotroph and thyrotroph. Those that do not stain for any hormone by immunocytochemistry

Dr P.J. Snyder has been a consultant to Novartis and Pfizer, and has received research funding from Novartis. Dr S.E. Mayson is an investigator in the ACCESS trial (Novartis) and COR-2012-01.
[a] Division of Endocrinology, The Warren Alpert Medical School, Brown University, 900 Warren Avenue, Suite 300, East Providence, RI 02914, USA; [b] Division of Endocrinology, Diabetes and Metabolism, Perelman School of Medicine, University of Pennsylvania, 12-135, 3400 Civic Center Boulevard, Philadelphia, PA 19104-5160, USA
* Corresponding author.
E-mail address: pjs@mail.med.upenn.edu

Endocrinol Metab Clin N Am 44 (2015) 79–87
http://dx.doi.org/10.1016/j.ecl.2014.11.001
0889-8529/15/$ – see front matter © 2015 Elsevier Inc. All rights reserved.

endo.theclinics.com

> **Box 1**
> **Classification of pituitary adenomas based on the combination of immunocytochemistry, biochemical testing, and clinical findings**
>
> - Classic: Pituitary adenomas that secrete hormonal products in sufficient quantities to cause characteristic signs and symptoms related to the hormone excess.
> - Subtle: Pituitary adenomas that secrete hormonal products that produce mild clinical manifestations related to the hormone excess.
> - Clinically silent: Pituitary adenomas that can be classified by immunocytochemistry and secrete hormonal products that can be detected by biochemical testing but do not cause clinical signs or symptoms.
> - Totally silent: Pituitary adenomas that can be classified by immunocytochemistry as arising from a specific anterior pituitary cell type but do not secrete a sufficient amount of their hormonal products to affect the serum concentration or urine excretion.

are called null cell, and those that stain for multiple hormones are called plurihormonal.
- Any type of pituitary adenoma can be silent, but a larger percentage of gonadotroph and null-cell adenomas and smaller percentage of lactotroph, somatotroph, and corticotroph are silent.

Gonadotroph adenomas account for 25% to 35% of pituitary adenomas overall[3–5] and 43% to 64% of silent adenomas.[3,6] Null-cell adenomas are nearly as common.[3] Clinically silent somatotroph adenomas account for up to 9%[4] and clinically silent corticotroph adenomas 2.9% to 5.7% of pituitary adenomas in surgical series.[7,8] Silent lactotroph adenomas occur in 1% to 2%[3] and silent thyrotroph adenomas less than 1%.[3,6,9] About 2% are plurihormonal.[3]

CLINICAL PRESENTATIONS

Silent pituitary adenomas are often detected as an incidental finding on MRI or when patients experience neurologic symptoms related to mass effect (**Table 2**). Pituitary hormone deficiencies occur in up to two-thirds[10]; however, in the authors' experience, they are not usually the presenting findings.

Progression of a nonfunctioning pituitary adenoma to one that is clinically apparent may occur. Several reports have described patients with known silent corticotroph adenomas who subsequently develop Cushing disease.[8,11–13]

Table 1
Types of silent pituitary adenomas based on immunocytochemistry

Adenoma Type	Immunostaining
Null cell	None
Gonadotroph	FSH, LH, α-subunit
Thyrotroph	TSH
Corticotroph	ACTH
Somatotroph	GH
Lactotroph	Prolactin
Plurihormonal	Multiple hormones

Abbreviations: ACTH, adrenocorticotropic hormone; FSH, follicle-stimulating hormone; GH, growth hormone; LH, luteinizing hormone; TSH, thyroid-stimulating hormone.

Table 2
Clinical presentations of silent pituitary adenomas

Presenting Feature	Frequency
Incidental finding on MRI	7.9%–37.5%[25,47]
Neurologic symptoms	
Visual field deficits	60.8%[14]
Extraocular muscle palsy	14.2%[14]
Headaches	9.7%–60.8%[10,14,47]
Hormonal deficiencies	
GH	35.8%–61%[10,14]
LH/FSH	40%[10,14]
TSH	35.8%[14]
ACTH	32.7%[14]
Diabetes insipidus	1.9%[10]
Pituitary apoplexy	3.7%–9.6%[14,47]

Abbreviations: ACTH, adrenocorticotropic hormone; FSH, follicle-stimulating hormone; GH, growth hormone; LH, luteinizing hormone; TSH, thyroid-stimulating hormone.
Data from Refs.[10,14,25,47]

DIAGNOSTIC EVALUATION

MRI is indicated to define both the size and extent of a silent pituitary adenoma. Extension into the sphenoid and cavernous sinuses can be seen in 14.2% to 16.9% and 19.2% to 33.2% of patients with nonfunctioning adenomas.[10,14] Humphrey visual field testing is indicated when the mass extends into the suprasellar cistern and elevates the optic apparatus.

All patients with nonfunctioning pituitary adenomas should undergo biochemical testing to evaluate for pituitary hormone excess. For those with clinically silent pituitary adenomas, biochemical testing can identify the mass as a pituitary adenoma and may identify the kind of adenoma by demonstrating excessive secretion of pituitary hormones.

Gonadotroph Adenomas

In a patient with a clinically nonfunctioning sellar mass, a gonadotroph adenoma can be detected preoperatively by the in vivo hypersecretion of intact gonadotropins and/or their subunits.

In men with a sellar mass:

- An elevated follicle-stimulating hormone (FSH) associated with low testosterone and luteinizing hormone (LH) that is not elevated is diagnostic of a gonadotroph adenoma.
- An elevated serum FSH (with or without elevated alpha subunit) has been reported in up to one-quarter of patients with gonadotroph adenomas[5,15,16]; an isolated elevated alpha subunit concentration occurred in 7%.[16]
- An elevated testosterone and LH, with or without an elevated FSH, is also diagnostic of a gonadotroph adenoma.
- An increase in LH beta subunit in response to synthetic thyrotropin-releasing hormone (TRH) is also diagnostic,[17] but TRH is not available in the United States.

In women with a sellar mass:

- Premenopause, FSH hypersecretion by a gonadotroph adenoma can result in ovarian hyperstimulation. Clinical manifestations include oligomenorrhea or amenorrhea and large ovarian cysts. Biochemical testing will reveal elevated FSH, normal or low LH, and markedly elevated estradiol.[18,19]
- After menopause, an elevated FSH concentration in the setting of a low or low-normal LH is highly suggestive of a gonadotroph adenoma.
- LH beta subunit response to synthetic TRH also occurs in women.[20]

Thyrotroph Adenomas

In a series of 63 patients with silent pituitary adenomas, 4 clinically euthyroid patients had staining for thyroid-stimulating hormone (TSH) β by immunocytochemistry and elevated serum TSH levels.[15]

Somatotroph Adenomas

Clinically silent somatotroph adenomas can be recognized preoperatively on the basis of an insulinlike growth factor 1 (IGF-1) concentration above the age-specific normal range. In a series of 100 consecutive patients with pituitary adenomas that were surgically excised, 24 had somatotroph adenomas immunocytochemically. Of these, 8, fully one-third, had an elevated IGF-1 concentration but no signs or symptoms of acromegaly and could therefore be considered to be clinically silent (**Table 3**).[4] They were recognizable as somatotroph adenomas before surgery even though they resulted in not even subtle clinical manifestations of acromegaly.

Corticotroph Adenomas

Preoperative testing also may help identify a sellar mass as a silent corticotroph adenoma before pathologic confirmation. Multiple microcysts are seen within the adenoma more often in patients with silent corticotroph adenomas than in those with adenomas causing Cushingoid features or other silent pituitary adenomas.[21] In a retrospective series, patients who had silent corticotroph adenomas had significantly higher preoperative mean serum adrenocorticotropic hormone (ACTH) concentrations compared with null-cell adenomas (46 vs 19 ng/L; normal = 5–27 ng/L), despite having similar serum cortisol levels.[22] Another case series of 12 patients with silent corticotroph adenomas reported acute adrenal insufficiency in 2 patients after resection of their tumors, suggesting that they had secreted cortisol excessively preoperatively.[23]

Table 3
Distinguishing clinically silent and totally silent somatotroph adenomas from those that are subtle or classic

Classification	Acromegalic Features	Serum IGF-1	GH Immunostaining
Classic	Typical	Elevated	Positive
Subtle	Mild	Elevated	Positive
Clinically silent	None	Elevated	Positive
Totally silent	None	Normal	Positive

Clinically silent adenomas cannot be recognized by a patient's appearance but can be identified by an elevated serum insulinlike growth factor 1 (IGF-1) concentration.
Adapted from Wade AN, Baccon J, Grady MS, et al. Clinically silent somatotroph adenomas are common. Eur J Endocrinol 2011;165(1):39–44.

MANAGEMENT

The management of a silent pituitary adenoma can include the following:

- Observation
- Surgical resection
- Radiation therapy
- Medical therapy

Initial Treatment

Observation

Close clinical and radiographic monitoring without specific treatment is an option for silent pituitary adenomas that are not causing neurologic symptoms. Case series of silent pituitary macroadenomas that are observed have reported clinical progression in 20% to 50% of subjects observed for 42 to 118 months.[24–26] Because of high rates of progression, monitoring by MRI is essential when the patient is observed only.

Surgery

Transsphenoidal surgery is the single best treatment option for silent pituitary adenomas that are causing neurologic compromise and could be considered for very large adenomas at risk for this complication. It is the only treatment that has a high likelihood of improving symptoms rapidly. In a study of 279 patients with visual deficits, vision improved in 50.6% and normalized in 39.4% after surgery.[27] Although recovery of pituitary hormonal function may occur after surgery, a meta-analysis of 58 studies found that fewer than one-third of patients had postoperative improvement.[28] The detection of hypopituitarism in a patient with a silent pituitary adenoma should prompt treatment with hormone replacement and not in itself be considered an indication for surgery.

Complications after the transsphenoidal resection of a silent pituitary adenoma are similar to other pituitary macroadenomas. Postoperative complications may include the following:

- New visual field deficits (3%)[28]
- Cerebrospinal fluid leak or fistula formation (3%)[28]
- Meningitis (1%)[28]
- Blood loss requiring transfusion (<1%)[27]
- Sellar hematoma requiring surgical drainage in 1%[27]
- New hypopituitarism (11%)[29]
- Transient (18.7%) or permanent (0.8%) diabetes insipidus[14]
- Death (<1%)[28]

Treatment of Residual or Recurrent Disease

After surgery, MRI can diagnose residual or recurrent adenoma. Patients with residual adenoma seen on postoperative imaging experience higher rates of adenoma progression during follow-up. In a meta-analysis of 1614 patients followed for 42 to 112 months after surgery, the recurrence rate was 46% for those with residual adenoma seen on postoperative imaging versus 12% for those without.[30] The 10-year recurrence-free survival rate after transsphenoidal surgery was 100%, 58.3%, and 23.1% for patients with silent pituitary adenomas who had no residual, intrasellar residual, and extrasellar residual detectable postoperatively.[31]

It has been proposed that silent corticotroph adenomas may be more aggressive than other silent pituitary adenomas, but published studies are conflicting.

A retrospective study of 33 silent corticotroph adenomas and 126 ACTH-negative adenomas followed for an average of 42 months found no significant difference in the rate of recurrence.[32] Another study reported comparable overall recurrence rates, although a higher rate of multiple recurrences was seen for silent corticotroph adenomas.[33] A more recent series of 75 silent corticotroph adenomas and 1726 hormone-negative adenomas noted increased cavernous sinus invasion and higher rates of progression and recurrence for silent corticotroph adenomas compared with hormone-negative adenomas of similar size.[22]

Radiation therapy

Radiation therapy administered postoperatively decreases the likelihood of growth or recurrence of a silent pituitary adenoma.[27,28,34,35] Because the clinical effects are delayed, radiation is not usually used as primary therapy. Sources of radiation can include x-rays from a linear accelerator, gamma radiation from ^{57}Co (gamma knife), or protons from a particle accelerator. Radiation can be delivered as a single high dose (ie, stereotactic radiosurgery) or in multiple small fractions. Fractionated radiation therapy can be used in most circumstances, but stereotactic radiosurgery is limited to the treatment of small adenoma remnants that are not in close proximity to the optic apparatus.

The benefits of postoperative radiation include the following:

- Improved 5-year recurrence-free survival in patients with residual adenoma demonstrable on postoperative imaging (100% treated vs 39.2% untreated).[27]
- Improved overall progression-free survival (93% treated vs 33% untreated at 15 years).[35]

Several studies have evaluated the effects of single-dose radiation in the treatment of silent pituitary adenomas. Following single-dose gamma radiation, three-quarters of patients in one study had a decrease in adenoma volume after a median follow-up of 80 months.[36] Another study reported a progression-free interval of 94% at 5 years and 76% at 10 years after a single dose of radiation.[37]

Although there are well-documented benefits of radiation therapy, side effects preclude the use of postoperative radiation for all patients with silent pituitary adenomas. The benefits of radiation are more likely to outweigh the risks when a significant adenoma remnant is demonstrable on postoperative imaging and the likelihood of regrowth is high. Fatigue, nausea, and headaches are short-term risks that can occur for up to a few months after radiation therapy.

Long-term risks of radiation therapy include the following:

- New pituitary hormonal deficiencies in up to 70% of patients 10 years or more after radiation therapy[36,38–40]
- Optic neuropathy in 0.8% of patients at 10 years[41]
- Secondary intracranial tumors affecting nearly 2% of patients at 20 years[41]
- Increased risk of stroke in both men and women[41]

Medical Therapy

Dopamine agonists, somatostatin analogs, and other medical therapies have been tried for silent pituitary adenomas with only limited success.

Several case series have evaluated the use of dopamine agonists in the treatment of silent pituitary adenomas in general and silent corticotroph adenomas specifically. Most studies report only modest reductions in adenoma size, although more pronounced shrinkage and improvements in neurologic deficits have occasionally been seen.[42,43]

Because some silent pituitary adenomas express somatostatin receptors,[44–46] somatostatin analogs have also been tried. In one study, patients with postoperative remnants were divided into 2 groups on the basis of a positive or negative octreotide scan. The 26 patients who had positive scans were treated with long-acting octreotide, whereas the 13 with negative scans were observed.[44] After 1 year, the adenoma remnant had increased in 54% of the patients who were observed but in only 19% of those treated with octreotide (19%); neither visual fields nor pituitary function differed between the 2 groups.[44]

SUMMARY

We propose here a new classification of pituitary adenomas based on function. The classic category refers to adenomas that result in obvious clinical manifestations of hormonal excess, and the subtle category to the less obvious. Clinically silent adenomas are those that cause measurable hormonal excess but no clinical manifestations. Totally silent adenomas can be recognized only by immunocytochemical staining. Silent adenomas are frequently detected as incidental findings on MRI or because of symptoms due to mass effect. Surgery is indicated for silent adenomas associated with neurologic compromise. Postoperative radiation therapy is effective to prevent and treat recurrences, but not all silent adenomas require radiation.

REFERENCES

1. Fernandez A, Karavitaki N, Wass JA. Prevalence of pituitary adenomas: a community-based, cross-sectional study in Banbury (Oxfordshire, UK). Clin Endocrinol 2010;72(3):377–82.
2. Raappana A, Koivukangas J, Ebeling T, et al. Incidence of pituitary adenomas in Northern Finland in 1992–2007. J Clin Endocrinol Metab 2010;95(9):4268–75.
3. Saeger W, Ludecke DK, Buchfelder M, et al. Pathohistological classification of pituitary tumors: 10 years of experience with the German Pituitary Tumor Registry. Eur J Endocrinol 2007;156(2):203–16.
4. Wade AN, Baccon J, Grady MS, et al. Clinically silent somatotroph adenomas are common. Eur J Endocrinol 2011;165(1):39–44.
5. Ho DM, Hsu CY, Ting LT, et al. The clinicopathological characteristics of gonadotroph cell adenoma: a study of 118 cases. Hum Pathol 1997;28(8):905–11.
6. Yamada S, Ohyama K, Taguchi M, et al. A study of the correlation between morphological findings and biological activities in clinically nonfunctioning pituitary adenomas. Neurosurgery 2007;61(3):580–4 [discussion: 584–5].
7. Horvath E, Kovacs K, Killinger DW, et al. Silent corticotroph adenomas of the human pituitary gland: a histologic, immunocytologic, and ultrastructural study. Am J Pathol 1980;98(3):617–36.
8. Baldeweg SE, Pollock JR, Powell M, et al. A spectrum of behaviour in silent corticotroph pituitary adenomas. Br J Neurosurg 2005;19(1):38–42.
9. Wang EL, Qian ZR, Yamada S, et al. Clinicopathological characterization of TSH-producing adenomas: special reference to TSH-immunoreactive but clinically non-functioning adenomas. Endocr Pathol 2009;20(4):209–20.
10. Ferrante E, Ferraroni M, Castrignano T, et al. Non-functioning pituitary adenoma database: a useful resource to improve the clinical management of pituitary tumors. Eur J Endocrinol 2006;155(6):823–9.
11. Ambrosi B, Colombo P, Bochicchio D, et al. The silent corticotropinoma: is clinical diagnosis possible? J Endocrinol Invest 1992;15(6):443–52.

12. Salgado LR, Machado MC, Cukiert A, et al. Cushing's disease arising from a clinically nonfunctioning pituitary adenoma. Endocr Pathol 2006;17(2):191–9.

13. Melcescu E, Gannon AW, Parent AD, et al. Silent or subclinical corticotroph pituitary macroadenoma transforming into cushing disease: 11-year follow-up. Neurosurgery 2013;72(1):E144–6.

14. Chen L, White WL, Spetzler RF, et al. A prospective study of nonfunctioning pituitary adenomas: presentation, management, and clinical outcome. J Neurooncol 2011;102(1):129–38.

15. Oppenheim DS, Kana AR, Sangha JS, et al. Prevalence of alpha-subunit hypersecretion in patients with pituitary tumors: clinically nonfunctioning and somatotroph adenomas. J Clin Endocrinol Metab 1990;70(4):859–64.

16. Snyder PJ. Gonadotroph cell adenomas of the pituitary. Endocr Rev 1985;6(4): 552–63.

17. Daneshdoost L, Gennarelli TA, Bashey HM, et al. Identification of gonadotroph adenomas in men with clinically nonfunctioning adenomas by the luteinizing hormone beta subunit response to thyrotropin-releasing hormone. J Clin Endocrinol Metab 1993;77(5):1352–5.

18. Castelbaum AJ, Bigdeli H, Post KD, et al. Exacerbation of ovarian hyperstimulation by leuprolide reveals a gonadotroph adenoma. Fertil Steril 2002;78(6):1311–3.

19. Djerassi A, Coutifaris C, West VA, et al. Gonadotroph adenoma in a premenopausal woman secreting follicle-stimulating hormone and causing ovarian hyperstimulation. J Clin Endocrinol Metab 1995;80(2):591–4.

20. Daneshdoost L, Gennarelli TA, Bashey HM, et al. Recognition of gonadotroph adenomas in women. N Engl J Med 1991;324(9):589–94.

21. Cazabat L, Dupuy M, Boulin A, et al. Silent, but not unseen: multi-microcystic aspect on T2-weighted MRI in Silent Corticotroph Adenomas. Clin Endocrinol 2014;81:566–72.

22. Jahangiri A, Wagner JR, Pekmezci M, et al. A comprehensive long-term retrospective analysis of silent corticotrophic adenomas versus hormone-negative adenomas. Neurosurgery 2013;73:8–17.

23. Lopez JA, Kleinschmidt-Demasters BK, Sze CI, et al. Silent corticotroph adenomas: further clinical and pathological observations. Hum Pathol 2004; 35(9):1137–47.

24. Dekkers OM, Hammer S, de Keizer RJ, et al. The natural course of nonfunctioning pituitary macroadenomas. Eur J Endocrinol 2007;156(2):217–24.

25. Karavitaki N, Collison K, Halliday J, et al. What is the natural history of nonoperated nonfunctioning pituitary adenomas? Clin Endocrinol 2007;67(6):938–43.

26. Sanno N, Oyama K, Tahara S, et al. A survey of pituitary incidentaloma in Japan. Eur J Endocrinol 2003;149(2):123–7.

27. Losa M, Mortini P, Barzaghi R, et al. Early results of surgery in patients with nonfunctioning pituitary adenoma and analysis of the risk of tumor recurrence. J Neurosurg 2008;108(3):525–32.

28. Murad MH, Fernandez-Balsells MM, Barwise A, et al. Outcomes of surgical treatment for nonfunctioning pituitary adenomas: a systematic review and meta-analysis. Clin Endocrinol 2010;73(6):777–91.

29. Roelfsema F, Biermasz NR, Pereira AM. Clinical factors involved in the recurrence of pituitary adenomas after surgical remission: a structured review and meta-analysis. Pituitary 2012;15(1):71–83.

30. Chen Y, Wang CD, Su ZP, et al. Natural history of postoperative nonfunctioning pituitary adenomas: a systematic review and meta-analysis. Neuroendocrinology 2012;96(4):333–42.

31. O'Sullivan EP, Woods C, Glynn N, et al. The natural history of surgically treated but radiotherapy-naive nonfunctioning pituitary adenomas. Clin Endocrinol 2009;71(5):709–14.
32. Ioachimescu AG, Eiland L, Chhabra VS, et al. Silent corticotroph adenomas: Emory University cohort and comparison with ACTH-negative nonfunctioning pituitary adenomas. Neurosurgery 2012;71(2):296–303 [discussion: 304].
33. Cho HY, Cho SW, Kim SW, et al. Silent corticotroph adenomas have unique recurrence characteristics compared with other nonfunctioning pituitary adenomas. Clin Endocrinol 2010;72(5):648–53.
34. Brochier S, Galland F, Kujas M, et al. Factors predicting relapse of nonfunctioning pituitary macroadenomas after neurosurgery: a study of 142 patients. Eur J Endocrinol 2010;163(2):193–200.
35. Gittoes NJ, Bates AS, Tse W, et al. Radiotherapy for non-function pituitary tumours. Clin Endocrinol 1998;48(3):331–7.
36. Gopalan R, Schlesinger D, Vance ML, et al. Long-term outcomes after Gamma Knife radiosurgery for patients with a nonfunctioning pituitary adenoma. Neurosurgery 2011;69(2):284–93.
37. Park KJ, Kano H, Parry PV, et al. Long-term outcomes after gamma knife stereotactic radiosurgery for nonfunctional pituitary adenomas. Neurosurgery 2011; 69(6):1188–99.
38. Dekkers OM, Pereira AM, Romijn JA. Treatment and follow-up of clinically nonfunctioning pituitary macroadenomas. J Clin Endocrinol Metab 2008;93(10): 3717–26.
39. Loeffler JS, Shih HA. Radiation therapy in the management of pituitary adenomas. J Clin Endocrinol Metab 2011;96(7):1992–2003.
40. Tsang RW, Brierley JD, Panzarella T, et al. Radiation therapy for pituitary adenoma: treatment outcome and prognostic factors. Int J Radiat Oncol Biol Phys 1994;30(3):557–65.
41. Erridge SC, Conkey DS, Stockton D, et al. Radiotherapy for pituitary adenomas: long-term efficacy and toxicity. Radiother Oncol 2009;93(3):597–601.
42. Lohmann T, Trantakis C, Biesold M, et al. Minor tumour shrinkage in nonfunctioning pituitary adenomas by long-term treatment with the dopamine agonist cabergoline. Pituitary 2001;4(3):173–8.
43. Garcia EC, Naves LA, Silva AO, et al. Short-term treatment with cabergoline can lead to tumor shrinkage in patients with nonfunctioning pituitary adenomas. Pituitary 2013;16(2):189–94.
44. Fusco A, Giampietro A, Bianchi A, et al. Treatment with octreotide LAR in clinically non-functioning pituitary adenoma: results from a case-control study. Pituitary 2012;15(4):571–8.
45. Pawlikowski M, Pisarek H, Kunert-Radek J, et al. Immunohistochemical detection of somatostatin receptor subtypes in "clinically nonfunctioning" pituitary adenomas. Endocr Pathol 2003;14(3):231–8.
46. Taboada GF, Luque RM, Bastos W, et al. Quantitative analysis of somatostatin receptor subtype (SSTR1-5) gene expression levels in somatotropinomas and non-functioning pituitary adenomas. Eur J Endocrinol 2007;156(1):65–74.
47. Nomikos P, Ladar C, Fahlbusch R, et al. Impact of primary surgery on pituitary function in patients with non-functioning pituitary adenomas–a study on 721 patients. Acta Neurochir 2004;146(1):27–35.

Cabergoline Use for Pituitary Tumors and Valvular Disorders

Renata S. Auriemma, MD[a], Prof Rosario Pivonello, MD, PhD[b], Lucia Ferreri, MD[b], Prisco Priscitelli, MD, PhD[a], Prof Annamaria Colao, MD, PhD[b,*]

KEYWORDS

- Pituitary adenoma • Prolactinoma • Acromegaly • Cushing's disease • Cabergoline
- Dopamine-agonists • Cardiac valve disease

KEY POINTS

- Cabergoline is widely used for the medical treatment of pituitary tumors, particularly those associated with hormone hypersecretion.
- In patients with Parkinson disease, the use of ergot-derived dopamine agonists, such as cabergoline, is associated with the risk of developing clinically relevant cardiac valve disease.
- In prolactinomas and acromegaly, cabergoline was not associated with an increased risk of significant valvulopathy, and no correlation has been shown between valvular abnormalities and cabergoline duration or cumulative dose.
- No systematic study has investigated the association between medical therapy with cabergoline and cardiac valvulopathy in patients with nonfunctioning pituitary tumors and Cushing disease.
- In patients requiring high doses of cabergoline (>3 mg/wk) for prolonged periods, echocardiography may be necessary to assess for valvular abnormalities, whereas patients receiving typical doses of cabergoline (1–2 mg/wk) likely may not require regular echocardiographic screening.

Dr A. Colao has been principal investigator of research studies from Novartis, Ipsen, Pfizer, and Lilly; has received research grants from Ferring, Lilly, Ipsen, Merck-Serono, Novartis, Novo-Nordisk, and Pfizer; has been occasional consultant for Novartis, Ipsen, and Pfizer; and has received fees and honoraria from Ipsen, Novartis, and Pfizer. R. Pivonello has been principal investigator of research studies from Novartis; has received research grants from Novartis, Pfizer, Viropharma, and IBSA; has been occasional consultant for Novartis, Ipsen, Pfizer, Viropharma, Ferring, and Italfarmaco; and received fees and honoraria for presentations from Novartis. Dr R.S. Auriemma, Dr L. Ferreri, and Dr P. Priscitelli have nothing to disclose.
[a] Ios-Coleman Medicina Futura Medical Center, Centro Direzionale, Naples 80143, Italy;
[b] Dipartimento di Medicina Clinica e Chirurgia, Sezione di Endocrinologia, University "Federico II", via Sergio Pansini 5, Naples 80131, Italy
* Corresponding author. Dipartimento di Medicina Clinica e Chirurgia, Sezione di Endocrinologia, University "Federico II", via Sergio Pansini 5, Naples 80131, Italy.
E-mail address: colao@unina.it

INTRODUCTION

The goals of medical treatment of pituitary tumors include[1] removal of the tumor; preservation of normal residual pituitary function; prevention of recurrence; restoration of normal hormonal secretion; relief from symptoms directly caused by hormonal excess; prevention of disabling long-term consequences; and reversal of the poor long-term outcome, particularly in acromegaly and Cushing disease. Hormonally active pituitary adenomas can be medically treated. The dopamine D2 receptor subtype is the pharmacologic target of dopamine agonists (DAs), such as bromocriptine and cabergoline (CAB), which are widely used for medical management of pituitary tumors. Effectiveness of CAB in pituitary tumors is summarized in **Table 1**.[2–6]

CURRENT CONTROVERSIES

Besides the indication for medical treatment of pituitary tumors, DAs are the first-line treatment for Parkinson disease (PD).[7] In recent years, increasing evidence has associated the use of ergot-derived DAs, such as pergolide and CAB, with the risk of cardiac valve disease in 29% to 39% of patients with PD,[8–10] usually treated with mean weekly doses up to 25 mg[11] and taking median cumulative doses ranging from 2600 to 6700 mg,[12] with the risk of valvular disease being significantly related to cumulative dose and treatment duration.[13] Moreover, DA use in PD has been found not to be associated with an increased risk of newly diagnosed heart failure.[14] In PD, DA-induced valvular abnormalities have been hypothesized to be mediated by the serotoninergic system, as DAs have been demonstrated to have high affinity for the serotonin receptor subtype 2B, which is abundantly expressed in heart valves and is known to promote mitogenesis.[15,16] CAB and pergolide are potent agonists of these receptors, whereas bromocriptine and lisuride have antagonistic properties.[16]

Whether treatment with CAB is associated with an increased risk of clinically relevant cardiac valve disease (CRVD) in patients with pituitary tumors is still debated. Most experience has been collected in patients with prolactinomas, whereas scant data have been provided to date about the risk of CRVD in patients with acromegaly on CAB. No data are available about a similar association between CAB therapy and CRVD in patients with clinically nonfunctioning pituitary adenoma (NFA), and only a study of Cushing disease[6] documented no development of cardiac valve insufficiency or worsening of previously diagnosed valve insufficiency in all patients but one, who

Table 1
Effectiveness of treatment with cabergoline on disease control and tumor shrinkage in pituitary tumors

Tumor Histotype	Reference No.	Control of Hormonal Hypersecretion, %	Tumor Shrinkage, %
Prolactin-secreting	2,3	100	96
GH-secreting	4	34 (monotherapy) 52 (combined to somatostatin analogs)	35
NFA	5	—	27.6
ACTH-secreting	6	40	50 (of CAB responders)

Abbreviations: CAB, cabergoline; GH, growth hormone; NFA, clinically nonfunctioning pituitary adenoma.
Data from Refs.[2–6]

experienced the progression from mild to moderate tricuspid regurgitation after 2 years of treatment.

CABERGOLINE AND CARDIAC VALVULOPATHY IN PROLACTINOMAS

Over the past 6 years, 17 independent studies[17–33] (**Table 2**) have investigated the effects of CAB on the development of CRVD in patients with prolactinomas. Five studies[17,21,25,30,32] demonstrated an increased prevalence of nonclinically relevant regurgitations, including mild mitral[32] and tricuspid regurgitation,[21,25,30,32] pulmonic insufficiency,[21] or enlarged mitral tenting area.[17] Twelve studies[17,19,20,22,24,26–31,33] reported a variable prevalence of CRVD, ranging from 2%[29] to 54%,[20] including moderate to severe mitral or tricuspid insufficiency; mild aortic regurgitation has been observed in 3 investigations.[26,29,32] Overall, these studies reported a median CRVD rate of approximately 4%, with the prevalence of CRVD ranging from 54%[20] to 0%.[18,21,23,32] Valvulopathy prevalence has been correlated with CAB cumulative dose in only 2 reports,[20,30] whereas the vast majority of studies have documented the safety of CAB on cardiac valves in hyperprolactinemic patients. Noteworthy, only 2 studies[28,32] prospectively investigated the effects of long-term treatment with CAB on valvulopathy in patients with prolactinomas. Both demonstrated no significant increase in the risk of CRVD after 24[28,32] and 60 months[32] of CAB. Moreover, the prevalence of trivial valvulopathy found in some studies[20,21,30,32,34] resulted not increased as compared with that reported in the general population.[35] The prevalence of mild aortic regurgitation has been found to range from 2.0%[29] to 3.9%,[27] and has been reported to be not higher than that described in the general population.[35] Two studies[20,30] described a high prevalence of significant valvulopathy after treatment with CAB. These studies documented moderate tricuspid regurgitation to occur in 40%[30] and 54%[20] of cases, respectively, and to be related to CAB cumulative dose. Particularly, we reported an approximately 3 times higher relative risk of developing moderate tricuspidal regurgitation in treated patients as compared with controls and de novo patients.[20] The prevalence of moderate valve regurgitation was found significantly higher in patients treated with a median cumulative dose greater than 280 mg (72%) than in those receiving lower doses (36%).[20] More recently, in a prospective study,[32] we demonstrated the safety of long-term CAB use up to 5 years on cardiac valvulopathy. In this study,[32] median cumulative dose of CAB at both 2-year (48 mg) and 5-year evaluations (149 mg) was lower than in our previous observation.[20] A recent cross-sectional study[33] investigating the prevalence of cardiac valvular abnormalities in 747 hyperprolactinemic patients treated with ergot-derived DA (601 receiving CAB at a median cumulative dose of 152 mg) reported moderate valvular stenosis or regurgitation to occur in 3.2% of patients.[33] No associations have been observed between cumulative DA doses and the age-corrected prevalence of any valvulopathy.[33] The difference in CRVD prevalence between patients with prolactinomas and those with PD might reflect the remarkable difference in CAB cumulative doses used in such patients. Indeed, in a large series of patients,[34] treatment with DA was found associated with an increased risk of CRVD only in patients with PD but not in hyperprolactinemic patients.

Tricuspid tethering area has been found significantly wider in patients treated with CAB than in controls and de novo patients.[20] As previously reported in patients with PD,[13,36] CAB may induce subclinical fibrotic alterations in valve architecture, predisposing to severe dysfunctions. Lancellotti and colleagues[17] described mitral leaflet thickening in approximately 6% of patients receiving CAB, and found that mitral tenting area, a quantitative index of valve restriction, was significantly higher in patients

Table 2
Effects of treatment with cabergoline on valvular heart disease in patients with prolactinomas: overview of literature

Author, Reference No.	No. of Patients	Age, y	CD, mg	TD, mo	CRVD, %	Valve	Relation with CD
Lancellotti et al,[17] 2008	102	51 ± 14	18–1718	12–228	2	Mitral (thickening)	No
Devin et al,[18] 2008	45	41 ± 10	146 ± 220	39 ± 29	0	—	No
Kars et al,[19] 2008	47	47 ± 1	363 ± 65	62 ± 5	15 (grade 3) 2 (grade 4)	Tricuspid and aortic	No
Colao et al,[20] 2008	50	36 ± 10	414 ± 390	16–250	54	Tricuspid	Yes
Walik et al,[21] 2008	44	42 ± 13	311	44.8	0	—	No
Bogazzi et al,[22] 2008	100	41 ± 13	279 ± 301	67 ± 39	7	—	No
Herring et al,[23] 2009	50	51 ± 2	443 ± 53	12–156	0	—	No
Vallette et al,[24] 2009	70	44	282 ± 271	55 ± 22	5.7	—	No
Nachtigall et al,[25] 2009	100	44 ± 13	253 ± 52	48 ± 4	0	—	No
Tan et al,[26] 2010	72	38 (31–49)	126	53	2.7	Aortic	No
Boguszewski et al,[27] 2012	51	42 ± 13	238.7 ± 242	12–52	3.9	Aortic	No
Delgado et al,[28] 2012	45	48 ± 1.8	401 ± 55	24	5	Mitral and tricuspid	No
Elenkova et al,[29] 2012	103	38 ± 10	174	46 ± 28	2	Aortic	No
Halperin et al,[30] 2012	62	37 ± 10.6	216.2 ± 306	51 ± 42	40	Tricuspid	Yes
Cordoba-Soriano et al,[31] 2013	32	39 ± 10	158	30–96	6.2	Tricuspid and aortic	No
Auriemma et al,[32] 2013	40	38.7 ± 12.5	48 149	24 60	2.5 (grade 1)	Aortic	No
Drake et al,[33] 2014	601	42	152	60–72	3.2	Mitral, tricuspid, and aortic	No

Abbreviations: CD, cumulative dose; CRVD, clinically relevant valve disease; TD, treatment duration.
Data from Refs.[17–33]

with mild valvulopathy than in controls. In the series by Kars and colleagues,[19] mitral and aortic calcifications, as well as leaflet thickening of the tricuspid valve also have been reported.

Altogether, the results of these studies do not support a clinically concerning association between the use of CAB for the treatment of hyperprolactinemia and cardiac valvulopathy in more than 1600 patients. Therefore, in patients requiring very high doses for prolonged periods, echocardiography may be necessary to assess for valvular abnormalities, whereas patients receiving typical doses of CAB (1–2 mg/wk) likely may not require regular echocardiographic screening.[37]

CABERGOLINE AND CARDIAC VALVULOPATHY IN ACROMEGALY

Over the past 6 years, 8 independent studies[38–45] (**Table 3**) have reported on the impact of CAB in patients with acromegaly. Only 2 studies[38,39] systematically investigated the effects of CAB on the development of CRVD in patients with acromegaly, whereas the remaining 6 studies[40–45] reported no change in echocardiographic findings,[40] no development of new valvular abnormalities,[41] or no data.[42–45] Moreover, patient series are not homogeneous across studies, as they have included acromegalic patients receiving either CAB monotherapy[38,39,42,45] and combined to somatostatin analogs[41,43] or pegvisomant.[40,44] Nonclinically relevant valve regurgitations have been reported in 26.2%[38] and 50.4%[39] of patients, and included mild mitral regurgitation in 19.0%[38] and 9.6%,[39] whereas mild tricuspid regurgitation accounted for 7.1%[38] and 23.5%[39] of cases. CRVD has been described in 9.5%[38] and 21.0%[39] of patients, respectively. Overall, these studies reported a CRVD rate of approximately 5%. CRVD prevalence has been found not to differ between acromegalic patients and healthy controls.[38,39] Interestingly, as previously shown in acromegaly,[46–50] in both studies aortic insufficiency was reported to be more prevalent (75%) as compared with regurgitation found in other valves (25%).[38,39] Moreover, in the study by Maione and colleagues,[38] 26 of 42 patients were longitudinally followed while on CAB. Prevalence of valvular regurgitations at baseline and of new valve regurgitation on CAB was similar between treated patients and controls. Similarly, in the study by

---

Table 3
Effects of treatment with cabergoline on valvular heart disease in patients with acromegaly: overview of literature

Author, Reference No.	No. of Patients	Age, y	CD, mg	TD, mo	CRVD, %	Valve	Relation With CD
Maione et al,[38] 2012	42	42	263	35	9.5	Mitral, tricuspid, and aortic	No
Lafeber et al,[39] 2010	119 (19 with acromegaly)	50.3 ± 14.7	277	115	11.3 (21 in acromegaly)	Tricuspid and aortic (aortic in acromegaly)	No

Abbreviations: CD, cumulative dose; CRVD, clinically relevant valve disease; TD, treatment duration.

Data from Moyes VJ, Metcalfe KA, Drake WM. Clinical use of cabergoline as primary and adjunctive treatment for acromegaly. Eur J Endocrinol 2008;159(5):541–5; and Casini AF, Vieira Neto L, Fontes R, et al. Aortic root ectasia in patients with acromegaly: experience at a single center. Clin Endocrinol (Oxf) 2011;75:495–500.

Lafeber and colleagues,[39] CRVD prevalence was found not significantly different between patients and controls.[39] In both studies,[38,39] the investigators concluded that valvular abnormalities are more likely to be related to acromegaly itself rather than to CAB. Indeed, acromegaly is reportedly associated with cardiac valve disease, and some studies[51–53] reported an increased prevalence of mitral and aortic valve regurgitation in patients with active disease.

Maione and colleagues[38] and Lafeber and colleagues[39] also reported leaflet thickening, mainly involving the mitral valve, with no significant impact on leaflet stiffening as compared with controls.[39] No restriction of valve leaflets and no reduction in their motility was observed in the CAB group.[38]

As in the vast majority of studies in prolactinomas, no significant correlation has been demonstrated between CAB cumulative and CRVD in acromegalic patients.[38,39]

SUMMARY

In patients with pituitary tumors treated with CAB, no evidence for a strong correlation between the treatment dose and/or duration and the development of CRVD has been provided to date. Moreover, the prevalence of nonclinically relevant valve regurgitation was not increased as compared with the general population. Altogether, these studies support the safety of treatment with CAB on cardiac valve disease, particularly in patients with prolactinomas and acromegaly. Nevertheless, in patients receiving high-dose treatment, echocardiography may be necessary to assess for valvular abnormalities. Further studies also are needed to extend and confirm these data in patients with NFA and Cushing disease.

REFERENCES

1. Colao A, Lombardi G. Growth-hormone and prolactin excess. Lancet 1998; 352(9138):1455–61.
2. Biller BM, Colao A, Petersenn S, et al. Prolactinomas, Cushing's disease and acromegaly: debating the role of medical therapy for secretory pituitary adenomas. BMC Endocr Disord 2010;10:10.
3. Gillam MP, Molitch ME, Lombardi G, et al. Advances in the treatment of prolactinomas. Endocr Rev 2006;27:485–534.
4. Sandret L, Maison P, Chanson P. Place of cabergoline in acromegaly: a meta-analysis. J Clin Endocrinol Metab 2011;96(5):1327–35.
5. Colao A, Di Somma C, Pivonello R, et al. Medical therapy for clinically non-functioning pituitary adenomas. Endocr Relat Cancer 2008;15(4):905–15.
6. Pivonello R, De Martino MC, Cappabianca P, et al. The medical treatment of Cushing's disease: effectiveness of chronic treatment with the dopamine agonist cabergoline in patients unsuccessfully treated by surgery. J Clin Endocrinol Metab 2009;94(1):223–30.
7. Nutt JG, Wooten GF. Diagnosis and initial management of Parkinson's disease. N Engl J Med 2005;353:1021–7.
8. Van Camp G, Flamez A, Cosyns B, et al. Treatment of Parkinson's disease with pergolide and relation to restrictive valvular heart disease. Lancet 2004;363: 1179–83.
9. Schade R, Andersohn F, Suissa S, et al. Dopamine agonists and the risk of cardiac-valve regurgitation. N Engl J Med 2007;356:29–38.
10. Zanettini R, Antonini A, Gatto G, et al. Valvular heart disease and the use of dopamine agonists for Parkinson's disease. N Engl J Med 2007;356:39–46.

11. Valassi E, Klibanski A, Biller BM. Potential cardiac valve effects of dopamine agonists in hyperprolactinemia. J Clin Endocrinol Metab 2010;95:1025–33.
12. Kars M, Pereira AM, Bax JJ, et al. Cabergoline and cardiac valve disease in prolactinoma patients: additional studies during long-term treatment are required. Eur J Endocrinol 2008;159:363–7.
13. Andersohn F, Garbe E. Cardiac and noncardiac fibrotic reactions caused by ergot- and nonergot-derived dopamine agonists. Mov Disord 2009;24:129–33.
14. Mokhles MM, Trifirò G, Dieleman JP, et al. The risk of new onset heart failure associated with dopamine agonist use in Parkinson's disease. Pharmacol Res 2012; 65:358–64.
15. Redfield MM, Nicholson WJ, Edwards WD, et al. Valve disease associated with ergot alkaloid use: echocardiographic and pathologic correlations. Ann Intern Med 1992;117:50–2.
16. Jahnichen S, Horowski R, Pertz HH. Agonism at 5-HT2B receptors is not a class effect of the ergolines. Eur J Pharmacol 2005;513:225–8.
17. Lancellotti P, Livadariu E, Markov M, et al. Cabergoline and the risk of valvular lesions in endocrine disease. Eur J Endocrinol 2008;159:1–5.
18. Devin JK, Lakhani VT, Byrd BF 3rd, et al. Prevalence of valvular heart disease in a cohort of patients taking cabergoline for management of hyperprolactinemia. Endocr Pract 2008;14:672–7.
19. Kars M, Delgado V, Holman ER, et al. Aortic valve calcification and mild tricuspid regurgitation, but no clinical heart disease after 8 years of dopamine agonist therapy for prolactinomas. J Clin Endocrinol Metab 2008;93:3348–56.
20. Colao A, Galderisi M, Di Sarno A, et al. Increased prevalence of tricuspid regurgitation in patients with prolactinomas chronically treated with cabergoline. J Clin Endocrinol Metab 2008;93:3777–84.
21. Wakil A, Rigby AS, Clark AL, et al. Low dose of cabergoline for hyperprolactinemia is not associated with clinically significant valvular heart disease. Eur J Endocrinol 2008;159:R11–4.
22. Bogazzi F, Buralli S, Manetti L, et al. Treatment with low doses of cabergoline is not associated with increased prevalence of cardiac valve regurgitation in patients with hyperprolactinemia. Int J Clin Pract 2008;62:1864–9.
23. Herring N, Szmigielski C, Becher H, et al. Valvular heart disease and the use of cabergoline for the treatment of prolactinomas. Clin Endocrinol (Oxf) 2009;70:104–8.
24. Vallette S, Serri K, Rivera J, et al. Long-term cabergoline therapy is not associated with valvular heart disease in patients with prolactinomas. Pituitary 2009;12:153–7.
25. Nachtigall L, Valassi E, Lo J, et al. Gender effects on cardiac valvular function in hyperprolactinaemic patients receiving cabergoline: a retrospective study. Clin Endocrinol (Oxf) 2009;72:53–8.
26. Tan T, Cabrita IZ, Hensman D, et al. Assessment of cardiac valve dysfunction in patients receiving cabergoline treatment for hyperprolactinaemia. Clin Endocrinol 2010;73:369–74.
27. Boguszewski CL, dos Santos CM, Sakamoto KS, et al. A comparison of cabergoline and bromocriptine on the risk of valvular heart disease in patients with prolactinomas. Pituitary 2012;15:44–9.
28. Delgado V, Biermasz NR, van Thiel SW, et al. Changes in heart valve structure and function in patients treated with dopamine agonists for prolactinomas, a 2-year follow-up study. Clin Endocrinol 2012;77:99–105.
29. Elenkova A, Shabani R, Kalinov K, et al. Increased prevalence of subclinical cardiac valve fibrosis in patients with prolactinomas on long-term bromocriptine and cabergoline treatment. Eur J Endocrinol 2012;167:17–25.

30. Halperin I, Aller J, Varela C, et al. No clinically significant valvular regurgitation in long-term cabergoline treatment for prolactinomas. Clin Endocrinol 2012;77: 275–80.
31. Córdoba-Soriano JG, Lamas-Oliveira C, Hidalgo-Olivares VM, et al. Valvular heart disease in hyperprolactinemic patients treated with low doses of cabergoline. Rev Esp Cardiol 2013;66(5):410–2.
32. Auriemma RS, Pivonello R, Perone Y, et al. Safety of long-term treatment with cabergoline on cardiac valve disease in patients with prolactinomas. Eur J Endocrinol 2013;169(3):359–66.
33. Drake WM, Stiles CE, Howlett TA, et al. A cross-sectional study of the prevalence of cardiac valvular abnormalities in hyperprolactinemic patients treated with ergot-derived dopamine agonists. J Clin Endocrinol Metab 2014;99(1):90–6.
34. Trifirò G, Mokhles MM, Dieleman JP, et al. Risk of cardiac valve regurgitation with dopamine agonist use in Parkinson's disease and hyperprolactinaemia: a multi-country, nested case-control study. Drug Saf 2012;35:159–71.
35. Singh JP, Evans JC, Levy D, et al. Prevalence and clinical determinants of mitral, tricuspidal, and aortic regurgitation (the Framingham Heart Study). Am J Cardiol 1999;83:897–902.
36. Antonini A, Poewe W. Fibrotic heart-valve reactions to dopamine-agonists treatment in Parkinson's disease. Lancet Neurol 2007;6:826–9.
37. Melmed S, Casanueva FF, Hoffman AR, et al. Diagnosis and treatment of hyperprolactinemia: an Endocrine Society clinical practice guideline. J Clin Endocrinol Metab 2011;96(2):273–88.
38. Maione L, Garcia C, Bouchachi A, et al. No evidence of a detrimental effect of cabergoline therapy on cardiac valves in patients with acromegaly. J Clin Endocrinol Metab 2012;97(9):E1714–9.
39. Lafeber M, Stades AM, Valk GD, et al. Absence of major fibrotic adverse events in hyperprolactinemic patients treated with cabergoline. Eur J Endocrinol 2010; 162(4):667–75.
40. Bernabeu I, Alvarez-Escolá C, Paniagua AE, et al. Pegvisomant and cabergoline combination therapy in acromegaly. Pituitary 2013;16(1):101–8.
41. Vilar L, Azevedo MF, Naves LA, et al. Role of the addition of cabergoline to the management of acromegalic patients resistant to long term treatment with octreotide LAR. Pituitary 2011;14(2):148–56.
42. Howlett TA, Willis D, Walker G, et al. Control of growth hormone and IGF1 in patients with acromegaly in the UK: responses to medical treatment with somatostatin analogues and dopamine agonists. Clin Endocrinol (Oxf) 2013;79(5):689–99.
43. Suda K, Inoshita N, Iguchi G, et al. Efficacy of combined octreotide and cabergoline treatment in patients with acromegaly: a retrospective clinical study and review of the literature. Endocr J 2013;60(4):507–15.
44. Higham CE, Atkinson AB, Aylwin S, et al. Effective combination treatment with cabergoline and low-dose pegvisomant in active acromegaly: a prospective clinical trial. J Clin Endocrinol Metab 2012;97(4):1187–93.
45. Moyes VJ, Metcalfe KA, Drake WM. Clinical use of cabergoline as primary and adjunctive treatment for acromegaly. Eur J Endocrinol 2008;159(5):541–5.
46. Casini AF, Vieira Neto L, Fontes R, et al. Aortic root ectasia in patients with acromegaly: experience at a single center. Clin Endocrinol (Oxf) 2011;75:495–500.
47. Savage DD, Henry WL, Eastman RC, et al. Echocardiographic assessment of cardiac anatomy and function in acromegalic patients. Am J Med 1979;67:823–9.
48. van der Klaauw AA, Bax JJ, Smit JW, et al. Increased aortic root diameters in patients with acromegaly. Eur J Endocrinol 2008;159:97–103.

49. Colao A, Grasso LF. Aortic root ectasia in patients with acromegaly: an emerging complication. Clin Endocrinol (Oxf) 2011;75(4):420–1.
50. Wiper A, Eisenberger M, McPartlin A, et al. Gross aortic root dilation in a young woman with acromegaly. Exp Clin Cardiol 2012;17(4):257–9.
51. Cable DG, Dearani JA, O'Brien T, et al. Surgical treatment of valvular heart disease in patients with acromegaly. J Heart Valve Dis 2000;9:828–31.
52. Ohtsuka G, Aomi S, Koyanagi H, et al. Heart valve operation in acromegaly. Ann Thorac Surg 1997;64:390–3.
53. Colao A, Spinelli L, Marzullo P, et al. High prevalence of cardiac valve disease in acromegaly: an observational analytical prospective case-control study. J Clin Endocrinol Metab 2003;88:3196–201.

Invasive, Atypical and Aggressive Pituitary Adenomas and Carcinomas

Prof Dr Aydin Sav, MD[a],*, Fabio Rotondo, BSc[b], Luis V. Syro, MD[c],
Antonio Di Ieva, MD, PhD[d], Michael D. Cusimano, MD, PhD[d],
Kalman Kovacs, MD, PhD[b]

KEYWORDS

- Aggressive pituitary adenoma • Atypical adenoma • Invasive adenoma
- Noninvasive adenoma • Pituitary carcinoma • Diagnosis

KEY POINTS

- Pituitary adenomas can be classified according to pathologic, radiological, or clinical behavior as typical or atypical, invasive or noninvasive, and aggressive or nonaggressive adenomas.
- World Health Organization classification categorizes pituitary adenomas as typical and atypical. Pathologic features of atypical adenoma are defined as a Ki-67 labeling index greater than 3%, and/or extensive p53 immunoreactivity.
- Invasive adenomas show pathologic or radiological signs of invasion to the cavernous or sphenoid sinuses, bone, or nasal mucosa.
- According to clinical behavior, a pituitary adenoma can be either aggressive or nonaggressive, and the use of biomarkers in differentiating aggressive adenomas has a limited place in determining the prognosis.
- Pituitary carcinomas are rare, show cerebrospinal and/or systemic metastasis, show a higher index of Ki-67 and p53 protein than aggressive adenomas, and they usually are resistant to radiotherapy.

Disclosures: The authors have nothing to disclose.
The authors are grateful to the Jarislowsky and Lloyd Carr-Harris Foundations for their support.
[a] Department of Pathology, Acibadem University, School of Medicine, Kerem Aydinlar Yerleskesi, Icerenkoy Mahallesi, Kayisdagi Caddesi, No: 32, Atasehir, Istanbul, Turkey; [b] Division of Pathology, Department of Laboratory Medicine, St. Michael's Hospital, University of Toronto, Toronto, Ontario, Canada; [c] Department of Neurosurgery, Hospital Pablo Tobon Uribe and Clinica Medellin, Medellin, Colombia; [d] Department of Neurosurgery, St. Michael's Hospital, University of Toronto, Toronto, Ontario, Canada
* Corresponding author.
E-mail address: murataydinsav@gmail.com

INTRODUCTION

Pituitary adenomas constitute 10% to 15% of intracranial neoplasms.[1] Although pituitary adenomas are benign, some of them are known to show aggressive clinical behavior, such as invading adjacent tissues and proliferating rapidly.[2] Invasion of surrounding structures by pituitary adenomas complicates complete resection and is an important cause for postoperative recurrence.[3] Biological markers for the aggressive nature of pituitary adenomas have been investigated, but none of them are widely accepted as being responsible for invasiveness.[4] Pathogenic mechanisms underlying pituitary adenoma formation, progression, and invasion remain poorly understood. Mutations in oncogenes and tumor suppressor genes (TSGs) that might be prognostic predictors or gene therapy targets are rarely found in pituitary tumors.[5] Thus, further investigation of new oncogenes and TSGs is needed. Pituitary carcinoma is restricted to tumors of adenohypophyseal cells that show cerebrospinal and/or systemic metastasis. They are rare and account for only 0.1% to 0.2% of pituitary tumors.[6] Their prognosis is poor and about 80% of these patients die within 8 years.[7]

ATYPICAL, INVASIVE, AND AGGRESSIVE PITUITARY ADENOMAS

Pituitary adenomas can be classified according to their pathologic features, radiological findings, or clinical behavior as typical or atypical, invasive or noninvasive, and aggressive or nonaggressive adenomas. The terminology aggressive has been used synonymously with invasive or atypical when evaluating pituitary adenomas and has produced different interpretations.[8] Clear definitions are therefore required.

According to the World Health Organization (WHO), pituitary tumors are classified as typical or atypical adenomas and pituitary carcinomas.[8] Pituitary adenomas that show higher mitotic activity, a Ki-67 labeling index (LI) greater than 3%, and/or extensive p53 immunoreactivity are considered atypical adenomas. Typical adenomas are tumors with monotonous cells and lack these findings. Pituitary carcinomas are defined when metastases are present even if they do not show common histologic malignant features such as higher mitotic activity.[9]

Aggressive adenoma has been used to define a high risk of recurrence or lack of therapeutic response. This pituitary tumor group advances to multiple recurrences[2] and is resistant to conventional treatment. These tumors are larger in size, faster in growth, or both.[9] Diverse potential biomarkers used in differentiating aggressive adenomas have not yet been fully validated.[10] So far, histopathologic biomarkers have yielded unconvincing results in predicting invasive adenomas.[11,12] Because of a lack of complete validation, correlation between polysialic neural cell adhesion molecule and pituitary tumor transforming gene with invasive potential seems to be unreliable.[13]

Invasive adenomas are considered tumors with proven growth to adjacent structures, such as the cavernous sinuses, bone, and sphenoid sinus.[14,15] Suprasellar extension is not considered a criterion of invasiveness. Invasion can be detected with preoperative MRI, during surgery, or with histologic demonstration of tumor spread to the dura, bone, or nasal mucosa.[16,17] MRI is the most practical common approach to classifying invasion and the Knosp grading system is widely used.[18]

Dural invasion detected by microscopic examination is common, therefore it is not regarded as a consistent indicator of aggressive tumor behavior.[16] The overall rate of invasion into the cavernous sinus is 35% and macroadenomas tend to invade more frequently than microadenomas.[16] Microscopy shows that dural invasion of pituitary adenomas occurs in about 64% to 85% of cases.[17] In spite of some controversies,[18] dural invasion ratio is higher in large adenomas than in small adenomas.[14]

According to their clinical behavior, pituitary tumors can be considered as aggressive or nonaggressive. Tumors that show a high rate of recurrence, demand repeated surgeries, and are resistant to conventional treatments are usually considered aggressive adenomas.[19,20]

Correlations between these classifications are not proportional. Pathologic findings do not always correlate with the radiological findings and clinical behavior. Some typical adenomas (Ki-67<3%) have an aggressive clinical behavior with high rates of recurrence and resistance to medical and surgical treatments. They can be either invasive or noninvasive at MRI. However, atypical adenomas do not always have an aggressive clinical behavior, and they can also be invasive or noninvasive. Not all invasive adenomas show the pathologic features that would be needed to be considered atypical adenomas and their clinical behavior can be nonaggressive. Furthermore, some noninvasive tumors can behave aggressively. Thus, the terms typical and atypical adenoma should refer only to pathologic features, the terms invasive and noninvasive adenoma should refer to radiological and surgical findings, and the terms aggressive and nonaggressive pituitary adenoma should refer to their clinical behavior.[21]

A newer classification proposed 3 subgroups based on radiological and surgical characteristics designating invasiveness and aggressiveness of tumors: noninvasive, invasive, and aggressive-invasive adenomas, in which aggressive-invasive adenomas showed a Ki-67 LI greater than 1%, mitotic activity greater than 2 out of 10 high-power field, and p53 expression.[19] However, despite large-scale pathologic, ultrastructural, and molecular studies, the relationship between aggressiveness and tumor type is still unresolved. Some specific pituitary adenoma histotypes are more prone to aggressive behavior; for example, sparsely granulated somatotroph adenomas, densely granulated lactotroph adenomas, acidophil stem cell adenomas, thyrotroph adenomas, sparsely granulated corticotroph adenomas, Crooke cell adenomas, silent subtype 3 adenomas, null cell adenomas,[20,21] densely granulated somatotroph adenomas, sparsely granulated lactotroph adenomas, densely granulated corticotroph adenomas, follicle-stimulating hormone/luteinizing hormone cell adenomas, and plurihormonal adenomas.[9]

PITUITARY CARCINOMAS

Pituitary carcinomas are defined as tumors of the pituitary showing cerebrospinal and/or systemic metastasis. They are rare (about 150 tumors published to date) and account for only 0.1% to 0.2% of pituitary tumors.[14] Whether or not extensive invasion of the brain by a pituitary tumor is a further criterion for carcinomas is a matter of controversy.[8] Most of these tumors secrete adrenocorticotropic hormone,[22] prolactin (PRL),[6,7] or thyroid-stimulating hormone.[23] Growth hormone–positive[24] and gonadotrophin-releasing tumors are very rare.[25] Pituitary carcinomas rarely arise from inactive adenomas, but mainly from invasive relapsing adenomas.[26] Because of prior surgery and/or radiation therapies, tumor and its connective tissue components and neighboring structures may be changed and give way to blood-borne and subarachnoid spread to cranial/spinal or extracranial systemic metastasis.[27] They show a higher Ki-67 LI and p53 oncoprotein level and a lower expression of p27 in primary tumor and in its metastases.[28] Ras mutations can be found in PRL cell carcinomas.[29] c-erbB-2 membrane staining and increased proliferating cell nuclear antigen index were shown not only in sellar tumors but also their metastases.[30]

Structural patterns of metastases commonly express similar features to primary tumors.[26] In a series of 7602 pituitary lesions, the incidence was found to be 0.12%, which were distributed as corticotroph cell carcinoma (n = 7), lactotroph cell carcinoma (n = 3), and somatotroph cell carcinoma (n = 2).[24,26] Their prognosis is generally poor,[31] although patients with long-term survival have been described.[32] One recent study found significantly worse overall survival in patients with pituitary carcinomas than in patients with invasive adenomas, reduced overall survival in patients 65 years of age or older, significantly better overall survival in women compared with men at 12 months, and no difference in survival between patients who received radiation therapy and those who did not.[33] Two reports recently analyzed the problems related to the diagnosis and biological behavior of pituitary tumors.[34,35]

SUMMARY

Invasive adenomas show pathologic or radiological signs of invasion to the cavernous or sphenoid sinuses, bone, or nasal mucosa. WHO classification categorizes pituitary adenomas as typical and atypical. Pathologic features of atypical adenoma are defined as a Ki-67 LI greater than 3% and/or extensive p53 immunoreactivity. The clinical behavior of pituitary adenomas can be either aggressive or nonaggressive. Specific adenoma subtypes are more prone to act destructively than other subtypes. Pituitary carcinomas are rare, show cerebrospinal and/or systemic metastasis, show a higher index of Ki-67 and p53 protein than aggressive adenomas, and they usually are resistant to radiotherapy.

REFERENCES

1. Asa SL, Ezzat S. The cytogenesis and pathogenesis of pituitary adenomas [review]. Endocr Rev 1998;19(6):798–827.
2. Kaltsas GA, Nomikos P, Kontogeorgos G, et al. Clinical review: diagnosis and management of pituitary carcinomas. J Clin Endocrinol Metab 2005;90:3089–99.
3. Oruckaptan HH, Senmevsim O, Ozcan OE, et al. Pituitary adenomas: results of 684 surgically treated patients and review of the literature. Surg Neurol 2000; 53:211–9.
4. Salehi F, Agur A, Scheithauer BW, et al. Biomarkers of pituitary neoplasms: a review (part II). Neurosurgery 2010;67:1790–8 [discussion: 1798].
5. Melmed S. Pathogenesis of pituitary tumors. Nat Rev Endocrinol 2011;7:257–66.
6. Scheithauer BW, Kurtkaya-Yapicier O, Kovacs KT, et al. Pituitary carcinoma: a clinicopathologic review. Neurosurgery 2005;56:1066–74.
7. Pernicone PJ, Scheithauer BW, Sebo TJ, et al. Pituitary carcinoma: a clinicopathologic study of 15 cases. Cancer 1997;79:804–12.
8. Lloyd RV, Kovacs K, Young WF Jr, et al. Pituitary tumors: introduction. In: DeLellis RA, Lloyd RV, Heitz PU, et al, editors. World Health Organization classification of tumours. Pathology and genetics of tumours of endocrine organs. Lyon (France): IARC Press; 2004. p. 9–13.
9. Saeger W, Lübke DK, Buchfelder M, et al. Pathohistological classification of pituitary tumors: 10 years of experience with the German pituitary tumor registry. Eur J Endocrinol 2007;156:203–16.
10. Grossman A. The 2004 World Health Organization classification of pituitary tumors: is it clinically helpful? Acta Neuropathol 2006;111:76–7.
11. Jaffrain-Rea ML, Di Stefano D, Minniti G, et al. A critical reappraisal of MIB-1 labelling index significance in a large series of pituitary tumours: secreting versus non-secreting adenomas. Endocr Relat Cancer 2002;9:103–13.

12. Sav A, Rotondo F, Syro LV, et al. Biomarkers of pituitary neoplasms [review]. Anticancer Res 2012;32(11):4639–54.
13. Zhang X, Horwitz GA, Prezant TR, et al. Structure, expression, and function of human pituitary tumor-transforming gene (PTTG). Mol Endocrinol 1999;13: 156–66.
14. Daita G, Yonemasu Y. Dural invasion and proliferative potential of pituitary adenomas. Neurol Med Chir (Tokyo) 1996;36(4):211–4.
15. Fahlbusch R, Buslei R. The WHO classification of pituitary tumours: a combined neurosurgical and neuropathological view. Acta Neuropathol 2006;111:86–7.
16. Scheithauer BW, Kovacs KT, Laws ER Jr, et al. Pathology of invasive pituitary tumors with special reference to functional classification. J Neurosurg 1986;65: 733–44.
17. Daita G, Yonemasu Y, Nakai H, et al. Cavernous sinus invasion of pituitary adenomas. Relationship between magnetic resonance imaging findings and histologically verified dural invasion. Neurol Med Chir (Tokyo) 1995;35:17–21.
18. Knosp E, Kitz K, Steiner E. Pituitary adenomas with parasellar invasion. Acta Neurochir Suppl (Wien) 1991;53:65–71.
19. Wierinckx A, Auger C, Devauchelle P, et al. A diagnostic marker set for invasion, proliferation, and aggressiveness of prolactin pituitary tumors. Endocr Relat Cancer 2007;14:887–900. http://dx.doi.org/10.1677/ERC-07-0062.
20. Mete O, Asa SL. Clinicopathological correlations in pituitary adenomas. Brain Pathol 2012;22:443–53. http://dx.doi.org/10.1111/j.1750-3639. 2012.00599.x.
21. Mete O, Ezzat S, Asa SL. Biomarkers of aggressive pituitary adenomas. J Mol Endocrinol 2012;49(2):R69–78. http://dx.doi.org/10.1530/JME-12-0113.
22. Zahedi A, Booth GL, Smyth HS, et al. Distinct clonal composition of primary and metastatic adrenocorticotrophic hormone-producing pituitary carcinoma. Clin Endocrinol (Oxf) 2001;55:549–56.
23. Mixson AJ, Friedman TC, Katz DA, et al. Thyrotropin-secreting pituitary carcinoma. J Clin Endocrinol Metab 1993;76:529–33.
24. Flitsch J, Lüdecke DK, Saeger W, et al. Dedifferentiation of a growth-hormone secreting pituitary adenoma to a non-secreting carcinoma. Exp Clin Endocrinol Diabetes 2005;113:S67 [abstract: 158].
25. McCutcheon IE, Pieper DR, Fuller GN, et al. Pituitary carcinoma containing gonadotropins: treatment by radical excision and cytotoxic chemotherapy: case report. Neurosurgery 2000;46:1233–40.
26. Lübke D, Saeger W. Carcinomas of the pituitary: definition and review of the literature. Gen Diagn Pathol 1995;141:81–92.
27. Waltz TA, Brownell B. Sarcoma: a possible late result of effective radiation therapy for pituitary adenoma. Report of two cases. J Neurosurg 1966;24:901–7.
28. Thapar K, Scheithauer BW, Kovacs K, et al. p53 expression in pituitary adenomas and carcinomas: correlation with invasiveness and tumor growth fractions. Neurosurgery 1996;38:765–71.
29. Cai WY, Alexander JM, Hedley-Whyte ET, et al. Ras mutations in human prolactinomas and pituitary carcinomas. J Clin Endocrinol Metab 1994;78:89–93.
30. Nose-Alberti V, Mesquita MI, Martin LC, et al. Adrenocorticotropin-producing pituitary carcinoma with expression of c-erbB-2 and high PCNA index: a comparative study with pituitary adenomas and normal pituitary tissues. Endocr Pathol 1998;9(1):53–62.
31. Dudziak K, Honegger J, Bornemann A, et al. Pituitary carcinoma with malignant growth from first presentation and fulminant clinical course: case report and review of the literature. J Clin Endocrinol Metab 2011;96:2665–9.

32. Landman RE, Horwith M, Peterson RE, et al. Long-term survival with ACTH-secreting carcinoma of the pituitary: a case report and review of the literature. J Clin Endocrinol Metab 2002;87(7):3084–9.

33. Hansen TM, Batra S, Lim M, et al. Invasive adenoma and pituitary carcinoma: a SEER database analysis. Neurosurg Rev 2014;37(2):279–85. http://dx.doi.org/10.1007/s10143-014-0525-y [discussion: 285–6].

34. Di Ieva A, Rotondo F, Syro LV, et al. Aggressive pituitary adenomas-diagnosis and emerging treatments. Nat Rev Endocrinol 2014;10:423–35. http://dx.doi.org/10.1038/nrendo.2014.64.

35. Syro LV, Builes CE, Di Ieva A, et al. Improving differential diagnosis of pituitary adenomas. Expert Rev Endocrinol Metab 2014;9(4):377–86.

Outcomes of Endoscopic Transsphenoidal Pituitary Surgery

Robert F. Dallapiazza, MD, PhD, John A. Jane Jr, MD*

KEYWORDS

- Endoscopic • Transsphenoidal • Pituitary • Cushing disease • Acromegaly
- Prolactinoma • Nonfunctioning macroadenoma • Hypopituitarism

KEY POINTS

- High rates of remission are achieved with endoscopic surgery in patients with Cushing disease, acromegaly, and medication-resistant prolactinomas; for nonfunctioning macroadenomas, there is a high rate of complete resection and improvement of vision.
- There are low rates of surgical complications including cerebrospinal fluid rhinorrhea, intracerebral hemorrhage, vision loss, and postoperative meningitis; sinonasal complaints are common, self-limited complications from transsphenoidal surgery.
- For secretory and nonfunctional tumors, failure to achieve biochemical remission or gross total resection (respectively) is largely determined by tumor invasion into surrounding structures.
- The theoretic advantage of endoscopic transsphenoidal surgery compared with microscopic surgery is that the endoscope provides a panoramic view allowing improved lighting and direct visualization of larger tumors.
- Despite the theoretic advantages of endoscopic surgery, evidence suggests that endoscopic and microscopic transsphenoidal surgery provide similar results if the surgeon is experienced; surgeon experience and tumor invasiveness are primary determinants of outcome, regardless of whether an endoscope or microscope is used for visualization.

INTRODUCTION

Advances Leading to Fully Endoscopic Transsphenoidal Surgery

The first reports of endoscopic-assisted transsphenoidal surgery were published in 1977 and 1978 for pituitary adenomas with significant extrasellar extension.[1] Jankowski and colleagues[2] reported the first fully endoscopic endonasal transsphenoidal surgery in 1992, which was subsequently expanded by Jho and Carrau[3]

The authors have nothing to disclose.
Department of Neurosurgery, University of Virginia, PO Box 800212, Charlottesville, VA 22908–0711, USA
* Corresponding author.
E-mail address: johnjanejr@virginia.edu

(an otorhinolaryngologist) in 1997. Multiple surgeons in the United States and Europe have contributed to the emergence and acceptance of this technique. The endoscopic technique allows dynamic, magnified, panoramic views, and angled scopes facilitate identification of the parasellar extensions not visualized by the microscope. Although the endoscope allows a greater portion of larger tumors to be removed under direct visualization, the lack of a speculum can hamper the free movement of instruments within the surgical field. Since its first reports in the literature, endoscopic transsphenoidal surgery has become an increasingly common method for removing pituitary tumors.

Surgical Method

There are several variations for endoscopic transsphenoidal surgery. Some surgeons access the sphenoid sinus through only one nostril, whereas others choose a binarial approach. Resecting part or all of the middle and superior turbinates can widen the surgical corridor in patients with narrow nasal cavities but risks sinonasal morbidity. The posterior nasal septum and rostrum of the sphenoid can be removed to various degrees to provide a single working corridor. In our practice, we use a binarial approach with partial posterior septectomy, wide anterior sphenoidotomy, and lateralization of the middle turbinates.[4]

Experience of the Surgeon

Most neurosurgeons are familiar with the use of the operating microscope for delicate microdissection. These skills are easily applied to microscopic transsphenoidal surgery. However, the endoscope is used less frequently as a surgical tool among neurosurgeons, which requires the development of a new set of skills, not only by the surgeon but also by their assistants. In transitioning from microscopic surgery to endoscopic surgery, several surgeons reported on the "learning curve" of the endoscopic method, which typically involves between 25 and 50 operations where the surgeon and team learn the nuances of the approach and adenoma dissection. Particularly useful in this process (and beyond) is a close partnership between pituitary surgeons and an otorhinolaryngologist who specializes in sinus surgery and endoscopic methods. Their expertise is especially important in patients with pre-existing sinus disease, septal perforations or deviations, and for large tumors where a skull-based reconstruction may be necessary.

OUTCOMES FOR REMISSION OF HORMONE-SECRETING TUMORS
Cushing Disease

Cushing disease (CD) is among the more challenging entities faced by neuroendocrinologists and pituitary surgeons. Diagnosis and treatment are made challenging because a significant number of patients have negative imaging despite advanced techniques. The goals of transsphenoidal surgery are remission of hypercortisolemia by complete removal of the adenoma while maintaining normal pituitary function.

Large series from experienced pituitary centers report overall biochemical remission rates in CD between 65% and 87% using a microscopic transsphenoidal approach.[5–9] In general, these series report that patients with MRI-negative adenomas and large, invasive tumors have lower rates of remission compared with patients with microadenomas and noninvasive macroadenomas.

There are few large series reporting the outcomes of endoscopic transsphenoidal surgery for CD (**Table 1**).[10–12] Many of the early reports include the outcomes of all types of pituitary adenomas and do not necessarily delineate MRI-negative CD or

Table 1
Endoscopic series for Cushing disease

Reference	n	Follow-up, m	Remission Criteria	Overall (%)	Micro (%)	Macro (%)
Berker et al,[10] 2014	90	32, 5–75	AM serum cortisol <5 1 mg DST	90	87	97
Starke et al,[11] 2013	61	28, 12–72	24-h UFC <20 AM serum cortisol <5	95	97	87
Wagenmakers et al,[12] 2013	86	71, 5–164	Basal serum cortisol <5 1 mg DST	72	83	94
Dehdashti et al,[13] 2008	25	17, 3–32	Normal 24-h UFC 1 mg DST	80	100	57
Frank et al,[14] 2006	56		AM serum cortisol <5 Normal 24-h UFC	68	68	68

Abbreviations: AM, morning; DST, dexamethasone suppression test; UFC, urinary free cortisol.
Data from Refs.[10–14]

invasive macroadenomas.[13–15] In 2013, Starke and colleagues[11] and Wagenmakers and colleagues[12] each reported large endoscopic transsphenoidal series in patients with CD with overall biochemical remission rates of 95% (at discharge) and 72%, respectively. Starke and colleagues[11] concluded that the endoscopic approach provided a similar remission rate compared with microscopic surgery and found no difference in the remission rate of MRI-negative CD, microadenomas, and macroadenomas. However, in this study the rate of remission of invasive tumors was not independently analyzed. Wagenmakers and colleagues[12] concluded that the dynamic visualization afforded by endoscopic approach allowed for more aggressive resection of invasive tumors, particularly those in the cavernous sinus. Nevertheless, the rate of biochemical cure was only 40%. In cases of MRI-negative CD Wagenmakers and colleagues[12] reported 60% remission in patients with MRI-negative CD that is comparable with previous microscopic series. One study compared microscopic and endoscopic surgery for CD and found no difference in the remission rate between these two methods.[16]

Many of microscopic series for CD have long-term follow-up and report recurrence rates up to 14%.[17] Starke and colleagues report a recurrence rate of 11% at 1 year, and Wagenmakers and colleagues report a rate of 16% at an average follow-up of 71 months. Although these recurrence rates are within the range of previously reported studies, future investigations of long-term efficacy of endoscopic transsphenoidal surgery for CD are warranted.

Proponents of the endoscopic approach note that it provides superior lighting of the surgical field, a dynamic view of the sella and surrounding structures, and the ability to use angled endoscopes to visualize recesses that cannot be seen in a microsurgical approach. However, the use of endoscopy sacrifices the stereoscopic vision afforded by the operating microscope. The latter point is particularly important in CD, because most tumors are small and contained within the sella. For these small tumors contained within the sella, the panoramic views of the parasellar spaces afforded by the endoscope are less relevant. Biochemical remission is best accomplished by dissecting the tumor circumferentially around the pseudocapsule to avoid leaving small remnants. Free movement of instruments within the operative field can be particularly challenging with the endoscopic technique. Although free movement can be accomplished with the endoscopic technique by progressively larger exposures (resection of the middle turbinates and larger removal of the nasal septum), this comes at the cost of potential nasal morbidity. Successful surgery requires careful exploration of the pituitary gland, an exploration that some surgeons believe is best accomplished using microsurgical techniques in which instruments can be used in an unencumbered manner. Nevertheless, there is little evidence comparing microscopic and endoscopic surgery in regards to biochemical remission rates or recurrence rate in patients with CD.

Acromegaly

Like CD, the primary treatment of acromegaly is transsphenoidal surgery, and the goal of surgery is to normalize growth hormone and insulinlike growth factor 1 levels by complete tumor resection. Unlike CD, somatotrophic adenomas do not present a significant diagnostic challenge and are typically larger and easily identified with preoperative imaging.

The rate of biochemical remission in large microsurgical series for acromegaly ranges from 30% to 70%.[18–22] In 2010, the international consensus guidelines applied more stringent criteria for remission of acromegaly, making comparisons of newly reported endoscopic series difficult with previous microscopic studies. Since then, four endoscopic transsphenoidal series have been published using the new criteria.[23–26] These studies report overall remission rates ranging from 46% to 70% with rates of remission ranging from 63% to 100% in microadenomas and 47% to 63% in macroadenomas (**Table 2**).[14,23–29] In these studies, cavernous sinus invasion was observed frequently (range, 25%–42% of cases), which likely contributes to the lower rate of remission in macroadenomas. Several of these studies found that remission rates were lower in invasive tumors. Hazer and colleagues[23] reported 54 cases of cavernous sinus invasion with a remission rate of 41%. Shin and colleagues[25] reported 14% remission of invasive tumors (Knosp grade 3 and 4) with surgery alone, and Jane and colleagues[26] reported 33% remission of Knosp grade 3 and 4 tumors (**Fig. 1** demonstrates the Knosp classification of pituitary adenomas). One study has directly compared microscopic with endoscopic surgery using the 2010 consensus guidelines in a contemporaneous series at a single center by two experienced surgeons, one microscopic and the other endoscopic. In this study, there was no significant difference in overall rate of remission (68% vs 71%), in remission of noninvasive tumors (87% vs 81%), or in invasive tumors (18% vs 45%).[30] The results of these studies suggest that despite a greater exposure and improved visualization of the endoscope the degree of invasion of the tumor plays a larger role than the mode of visualization (endoscope vs microscope).

Prolactinomas

The first-line treatment of these tumors is medical therapy with dopamine agonists. These medications normalize prolactin levels and decrease tumor volumes in approximately 80% of patients.[31,32] In those patients who are medically nonresponsive or cannot tolerate medical therapy, transsphenoidal surgery is indicated.

Most of the data for endoscopic transsphenoidal surgery for prolactinomas come from large, single-institutional studies that report the results of all tumor types (**Table 3**). In 2006, Frank and colleagues[14] reported on 66 patients with prolactinomas who underwent endoscopic surgery. The overall rate of biochemical remission was 76% in this study, and the rate of remission varied according to tumor invasion. In microadenomas the remission rate was 86%, for noninvasive macroadenomas the rate was 82%, and for invasive macroadenomas it was 37%.[14] In 2008, Dehdashti and colleagues[13] reported the results of 25 cases and achieved endocrinologic

Table 2 Endoscopic transsphenoidal series for acromegaly						
Reference	n	Follow-up, m	Remission Criteria	Overall (%)	Micro (%)	Macro (%)
Hazer et al,[23] 2013	214	34	Normal IGF GH <0.4 ng/mL after OGGT Random GH <1.0 ng/mL	63	63	63
Shin et al,[25] 2013	53	30, 3–128	Normal IGF GH <0.4 ng/mL after OGGT Random GH <1.0 ng/mL	51	83	47
Jane Jr et al,[26] 2011	60	22, 2–68	Normal IGF GH <0.4 ng/mL after OGGT Random GH <1.0 ng/mL	70	100	61
Hofstetter et al,[24] 2010	24	23, 2–74	Normal IGF GH <0.4 ng/mL after OGGT Random GH <1.0 ng/mL	46	—	—
Gondim et al,[29] 2010	67		Normal IGF GH <1 ng/mL after OGGT	75	86	72
Campbell et al,[27] 2010	26	25, 3–60	Normal IGF GH <1 ng/mL after OGGT Random GH <2.5 µg/L	58	75	54
Frank et al,[14] 2006	83		Normal IGF GH <1 ng/mL after OGGT Random GH <2.5 µg/L	73	86	69
Cappabianca et al,[28] 2002	36		Normal IGF GH <1 ng/mL after OGGT Random GH <2.5 µg/L	64	83	60

Abbreviations: GH, growth hormone; IGF, insulinlike growth factor; OGGT, oral glucose tolerance test.
Data from Refs.[14,23–29]

remission 96% of patients with microadenomas and noninvasive macroadenomas, but none of their patients with invasive tumors achieved remission. Yano and colleagues[33] published similar results in 2009 with endocrinologic remission in 94% of microadenomas and 42% of macroadenomas. One study by Cho and Liau[34] in 2002 compared microsurgery with endoscopic surgery in 44 patients with prolactinomas. They found no difference in remission rates between these two methods (66% vs 75%).

Nonfunctioning Macroadenomas

Like CD and acromegaly, the first-line treatment of nonfunctioning macroadenoma (NFM) is transsphenoidal surgery. However, the goal of surgery for NFM is more often to decompress the optic apparatus, maintain normal pituitary function, and prevent symptomatic recurrence. Unlike biochemical remission of CD and acromegaly, this does not necessarily require complete tumor removal.

As with prolactinomas, most of the data regarding endoscopic surgery for NFM are from single institutional studies that report outcomes for all tumor types. From these studies the rate of complete resection varies from 43% to 96%. Frank and colleagues[14] reported 173 cases with a rate of total resection of 77%. Gondim and colleagues[35] reported similar results in 2010 achieving complete resection in 71% of 135 patients. Yano and colleagues[33] had a slightly lower rate of complete

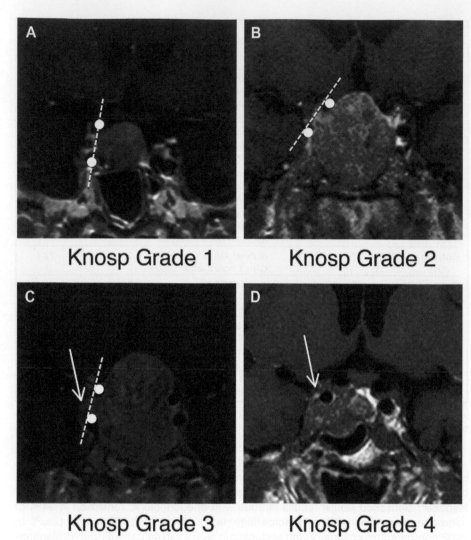

Fig. 1. Pituitary adenoma grading using the Knosp scale. (*A*) Knosp grade 1 adenomas do not extend beyond the midline of the intracavernous internal carotid artery (ICA). ICA is marked with *white circles* and midline is drawn with a *dashed yellow line*. (*B*) Knosp grade 2 adenomas extend to the lateral ICA tangential, but do not extend beyond. The ICA is marked with *white circles*, and the lateral ICA tangential line is marked with a *dashed yellow line*. (*C*) Knosp grade 3 adenomas extend laterally beyond the lateral ICA tangential line. ICA and lateral tangential line are marked as in *B*, and the *arrow* shows lateral extension. (*D*) Knosp grade 4 adenomas completely surround the intracavernous ICA (*arrow*).

resection (56%) in their study of 131 patients, and Dehdashti and colleagues[13] had a slightly higher rate at 88%. In this study, they noted that 10 patients had cavernous sinus invasion, and these tumors were incompletely removed. One study presents results from a pure series of NFM operated by endoscopic transsphenoidal surgery, which focuses on extremely large tumors with significant suprasellar extension. In this study the rate of gross total resection was 47%.[36] There are several

Table 3					
Endoscopic transsphenoidal results for prolactinomas					
Reference	n	Remission Criteria	Overall	Micro (%)	Macro (%)
Frank et al,[14] 2006	83	Normal prolactin	76	86	82/37[a]
Dehdashti et al,[13] 2008	25	Prolactin <20 ng/mL	88	100	91/0[a]
Yano et al,[33] 2009	29	Normal prolactin	72	94	42
Cho and Liau,[34] 2002	22	Normal prolactin	66	—	—

[a] These studies reported rates of remission for patients with noninvasive/invasive macroadenomas.
Data from Refs.[13,14,33,34]

large series that report outcomes from microsurgical transsphenoidal surgery for NFM. In these studies, rates of complete resection range from 28% to 83%.[37–43] One study directly compared microscopic with endoscopic surgery in noninvasive NFM and found no difference in the rate of complete resection using these two methods.[44]

Long-term follow-up is available from several microsurgical series. These series suggest recurrence rates ranging from 6% to 21%.[37,45] However, none of the single institutional reports of endoscopic series discuss long-term outcomes or rates of tumor recurrence. We reviewed our outcomes in patients undergoing endoscopic surgery for NFM who had a minimum of 5 years of clinical and radiographic follow-up. In this study, complete resection was accomplished in 71% of patients based on MRI at 1 year. Of the patients who had apparent gross total resection, 12% had imaging evidence of recurrence at a mean time of 53 months after surgery. In patients with a subtotal resection, 52% of patients had evidence of regrowth at a mean time of 36 months.[46] These findings highlight the need for long-term surveillance in patients with NFM.

Progressive visual loss is a hallmark symptom of NFM when growth extends into the suprasellar space and causes compression of the optic chiasm. Visual deficits are reported in 50% to 70% of patients with NFM.[13,35,37,39,40,43] In an overwhelming number of cases, surgical decompression improves or stabilizes visual function regardless of the surgical technique. Dehdashti and colleagues[13] reported that 54% of patients had complete improvement, 39% had partial improvement, and 9% had no change. There are few reports of worsening vision after either microscopic or endoscopic surgery. In many of these reported cases, there were hemorrhagic complications postoperatively, and very few patients had permanent visual worsening.[28,35]

OPERATIVE COMPLICATIONS

Among the serious postoperative complications reported after endoscopic transsphenoidal surgery, cerebrospinal fluid leak is the most common ranging from 1% to 6% of cases.[3,11,13–15,24,26,34] Operative mortalities, postoperative hemorrhages, and meningitis are rare, reported in less than 1% of cases (Table 4). This is not significantly different from microscopic series.

Postoperative Hypopituitarism

Newly diagnosed, postoperative hypopituitarism is a well-known complication of pituitary surgery. After surgery many patients require pituitary hormone replacement medications; however, most of these patients are able to discontinue these medications in the 2 to 6 months after surgery. Permanent diabetes insipidus is reported in

Table 4	
Complication rates from endoscopic transsphenoidal surgery	
Complication	**Rate (%)**
Surgical	
Cerebrospinal fluid leak	2%–16%
Meningitis	<1%
Hematoma	<1%
Mortality	<1%
Endocrinologic	
Diabetes insipidus	1%–5%
Anterior pituitary	3%–14%
Nasal	
Sinusitis	10%–30%
Epistaxis	1%–10%

1% to 5% of cases of endoscopic transsphenoidal surgery for pituitary adenomas. New anterior pituitary insufficiency is observed in 3% to 14% of cases with most series reporting 5% to 7% (see **Table 4**).[10–12,23,25,26,28,29] Improved visualization of the normal pituitary gland during endoscopic surgery may allow for better preservation of the remaining gland and lead to better endocrinologic results. Nevertheless, evidence of this theory has not been rigorously studied.

Nasal Outcomes

Postoperative sinonasal complaints are common in patients undergoing transsphenoidal surgery. These include nasal congestion, altered taste and/or smell, nasal crusting, septal perforations, and sinusitis. Fortunately, most of these symptoms are self-limiting and resolve within the first few months after surgery. More serious complications, such as recurrent sinusitis and postoperative epistaxis, are reported less frequently but may require further surgical treatment. Some authors believe that endoscopic surgery causes less trauma to the nasal cavity because it does not require the submucosal dissection, placement of intranasal retractors, or postoperative nasal packing that is standard in microscopic transsphenoidal surgery. However, endoscopic surgery does require the repetitive passage of instruments through the nasal cavity, which could cause trauma to the nasal mucosa and endonasal structures. Some studies cite a decreased incidence of sinonasal complaints following endoscopic surgery compared with previous microsurgical series.[14,28] However, few studies conclusively show that one approach is superior to the other in terms of sinonasal complaints.

SUMMARY

Endoscopic transsphenoidal surgery is an increasingly common method for resecting pituitary adenomas. Despite the theoretic and real advantages of the endoscopic technique, published reports have not proved superiority. Surgical remission of secretory adenomas and extent of resection of NFM likely relates more to individual surgeon experience and the degree of invasion of the tumor. Further studies are necessary to directly compare outcomes of endoscopic surgery with traditional microsurgical techniques. Furthermore, few studies report long-term outcomes from endoscopic surgery.

REFERENCES

1. Apuzzo ML, Heifetz MD, Weiss MH, et al. Neurosurgical endoscopy using the side-viewing telescope. J Neurosurg 1977;46(3):398–400.
2. Jankowski R, Auque J, Simon C, et al. Endoscopic pituitary tumor surgery. Laryngoscope 1992;102(2):198–202.
3. Jho HD, Carrau RL. Endoscopic endonasal transsphenoidal surgery: experience with 50 patients. J Neurosurg 1997;87(1):44–51.
4. Monteith SJ, Starke RM, Jane JA Jr, et al. Use of the histological pseudocapsule in surgery for Cushing disease: rapid postoperative cortisol decline predicting complete tumor resection. J Neurosurg 2012;116(4):721–7.
5. De Tommasi C, Vance ML, Okonkwo DO, et al. Surgical management of adrenocorticotropic hormone-secreting macroadenomas: outcome and challenges in patients with Cushing's disease or Nelson's syndrome. J Neurosurg 2005; 103(5):825–30.
6. Hammer GD, Tyrrell JB, Lamborn KR, et al. Transsphenoidal microsurgery for Cushing's disease: initial outcome and long-term results. J Clin Endocrinol Metab 2004;89(12):6348–57.
7. Oldfield EH. Surgical management of Cushing's disease: a personal perspective. Clin Neurosurg 2011;58:13–26.
8. Pouratian N, Prevedello DM, Jagannathan J, et al. Outcomes and management of patients with Cushing's disease without pathological confirmation of tumor resection after transsphenoidal surgery. J Clin Endocrinol Metab 2007;92(9): 3383–8.
9. Prevedello DM, Pouratian N, Sherman J, et al. Management of Cushing's disease: outcome in patients with microadenoma detected on pituitary magnetic resonance imaging. J Neurosurg 2008;109(4):751–9.
10. Berker M, Isikay I, Berker D, et al. Early promising results for the endoscopic surgical treatment of Cushing's disease. Neurosurg Rev 2014;37(1):105–14.
11. Starke RM, Reames DL, Chen CJ, et al. Endoscopic transsphenoidal surgery for Cushing disease: techniques, outcomes, and predictors of remission. Neurosurgery 2013;72(2):240–7 [discussion: 247].
12. Wagenmakers MA, Boogaarts HD, Roerink SH, et al. Endoscopic transsphenoidal pituitary surgery: a good and safe primary treatment option for Cushing's disease, even in case of macroadenomas or invasive adenomas. Eur J Endocrinol 2013; 169(3):329–37.
13. Dehdashti AR, Ganna A, Karabatsou K, et al. Pure endoscopic endonasal approach for pituitary adenomas: early surgical results in 200 patients and comparison with previous microsurgical series. Neurosurgery 2008;62(5):1006–15 [discussion: 1015–7].
14. Frank G, Pasquini E, Farneti G, et al. The endoscopic versus the traditional approach in pituitary surgery. Neuroendocrinology 2006;83(3–4):240–8.
15. Netea-Maier RT, van Lindert EJ, den Heijer M, et al. Transsphenoidal pituitary surgery via the endoscopic technique: results in 35 consecutive patients with Cushing's disease. Eur J Endocrinol 2006;154(5):675–84.
16. Alahmadi H, Cusimano MD, Woo K, et al. Impact of technique on Cushing disease outcome using strict remission criteria. Can J Neurol Sci 2013;40(3): 334–41.
17. Shimon I, Ram Z, Cohen ZR, et al. Transsphenoidal surgery for Cushing's disease: endocrinological follow-up monitoring of 82 patients. Neurosurgery 2002; 51(1):57–61 [discussion: 61–2].

18. Beauregard C, Truong U, Hardy J, et al. Long-term outcome and mortality after transsphenoidal adenomectomy for acromegaly. Clin Endocrinol 2003;58(1): 86–91.

19. Kaltsas GA, Isidori AM, Florakis D, et al. Predictors of the outcome of surgical treatment in acromegaly and the value of the mean growth hormone day curve in assessing postoperative disease activity. J Clin Endocrinol Metab 2001; 86(4):1645–52.

20. Ludecke DK, Abe T. Transsphenoidal microsurgery for newly diagnosed acromegaly: a personal view after more than 1,000 operations. Neuroendocrinology 2006;83(3–4):230–9.

21. Nomikos P, Buchfelder M, Fahlbusch R. The outcome of surgery in 668 patients with acromegaly using current criteria of biochemical 'cure'. Eur J Endocrinol 2005;152(3):379–87.

22. Shimon I, Cohen ZR, Ram Z, et al. Transsphenoidal surgery for acromegaly: endocrinological follow-up of 98 patients. Neurosurgery 2001;48(6):1239–43 [discussion: 1244–5].

23. Hazer DB, Isik S, Berker D, et al. Treatment of acromegaly by endoscopic transsphenoidal surgery: surgical experience in 214 cases and cure rates according to current consensus criteria. J Neurosurg 2013;119(6):1467–77.

24. Hofstetter CP, Mannaa RH, Mubita L, et al. Endoscopic endonasal transsphenoidal surgery for growth hormone-secreting pituitary adenomas. Neurosurg Focus 2010;29(4):E6.

25. Shin SS, Tormenti MJ, Paluzzi A, et al. Endoscopic endonasal approach for growth hormone secreting pituitary adenomas: outcomes in 53 patients using 2010 consensus criteria for remission. Pituitary 2013;16(4):435–44.

26. Jane JA Jr, Starke RM, Elzoghby MA, et al. Endoscopic transsphenoidal surgery for acromegaly: remission using modern criteria, complications, and predictors of outcome. J Clin Endocrinol Metab 2011;96(9):2732–40.

27. Campbell PG, Kenning E, Andrews DW, et al. Outcomes after a purely endoscopic transsphenoidal resection of growth hormone-secreting pituitary adenomas. Neurosurg Focus 2010;29(4):E5.

28. Cappabianca P, Cavallo LM, Colao A, et al. Surgical complications associated with the endoscopic endonasal transsphenoidal approach for pituitary adenomas. J Neurosurg 2002;97(2):293–8.

29. Gondim JA, Almeida JP, de Albuquerque LA, et al. Pure endoscopic transsphenoidal surgery for treatment of acromegaly: results of 67 cases treated in a pituitary center. Neurosurg Focus 2010;29(4):E7.

30. Starke RM, Raper DM, Payne SC, et al. Endoscopic vs microsurgical transsphenoidal surgery for acromegaly: outcomes in a concurrent series of patients using modern criteria for remission. J Clin Endocrinol Metab 2013;98(8):3190–8.

31. Colao A, Di Sarno A, Landi ML, et al. Long-term and low-dose treatment with cabergoline induces macroprolactinoma shrinkage. J Clin Endocrinol Metab 1997;82(11):3574–9.

32. Colao A, Di Sarno A, Sarnacchiaro F, et al. Prolactinomas resistant to standard dopamine agonists respond to chronic cabergoline treatment. J Clin Endocrinol Metab 1997;82(3):876–83.

33. Yano S, Kawano T, Kudo M, et al. Endoscopic endonasal transsphenoidal approach through the bilateral nostrils for pituitary adenomas. Neurol Med Chir 2009;49(1):1–7.

34. Cho DY, Liau WR. Comparison of endonasal endoscopic surgery and sublabial microsurgery for prolactinomas. Surg Neurol 2002;68(6):371–5 [discussion: 375–6]

35. Gondim JA, Almeida JP, Albuquerque LA, et al. Endoscopic endonasal approach for pituitary adenoma: surgical complications in 301 patients. Pituitary 2011; 14(2):174–83.
36. Nakao N, Itakura T. Surgical outcome of the endoscopic endonasal approach for non-functioning giant pituitary adenoma. J Clin Neurosci 2011;18(1):71–5.
37. Comtois R, Beauregard H, Somma M, et al. The clinical and endocrine outcome to trans-sphenoidal microsurgery of nonsecreting pituitary adenomas. Cancer 1991;68(4):860–6.
38. Ebersold MJ, Laws ER Jr, Scheithauer BW, et al. Pituitary apoplexy treated by transsphenoidal surgery. A clinicopathological and immunocytochemical study. J Neurosurg 1983;58(3):315–20.
39. Ferrante E, Ferraroni M, Castrignano T, et al. Non-functioning pituitary adenoma database: a useful resource to improve the clinical management of pituitary tumors. Eur J Endocrinol 2006;155(6):823–9.
40. Greenman Y, Ouaknine G, Veshchev I, et al. Postoperative surveillance of clinically nonfunctioning pituitary macroadenomas: markers of tumour quiescence and regrowth. Clin Endocrinol 2003;58(6):763–9.
41. Losa M, Mortini P, Barzaghi R, et al. Early results of surgery in patients with nonfunctioning pituitary adenoma and analysis of the risk of tumor recurrence. J Neurosurg 2008;108(3):525–32.
42. Woollons AC, Hunn MK, Rajapakse YR, et al. Non-functioning pituitary adenomas: indications for postoperative radiotherapy. Clin Endocrinol 2000; 53(6):713–7.
43. Chang EF, Zada G, Kim S, et al. Long-term recurrence and mortality after surgery and adjuvant radiotherapy for nonfunctional pituitary adenomas. J Neurosurg 2008;108(4):736–45.
44. Dallapiazza R, Bond AE, Grober Y, et al. Retrospective analysis of a concurrent series of microscopic versus endoscopic transsphenoidal surgeries for Knosp Grades 0-2 nonfunctioning pituitary macroadenomas at a single institution. J Neurosurg 2014;121(3):511–7.
45. Zhang X, Fei Z, Zhang J, et al. Management of nonfunctioning pituitary adenomas with suprasellar extensions by transsphenoidal microsurgery. Surg Neurol 1999;52(4):380–5.
46. Dallapiazza RF, Grober Y, Starke RM, et al. Long-term results of endonasal endoscopic transsphenoidal resection of nonfunctioning pituitary macroadenomas. Neurosurgery 2014. [Epub ahead of print].

Efficacy and Complications of Pituitary Irradiation

Georgia Ntali, MD, PhD, Niki Karavitaki, MSc, PhD, FRCP*

KEYWORDS

• Pituitary tumor • Pituitary radiotherapy • Hypopituitarism

KEY POINTS

• Radiation therapy is widely used in the management of intracranial (including sellar and parasellar) and systemic disorders.

• The place radiation therapy has in the management algorithm of pituitary tumors depends on the type of tumor, and it is usually recommended postoperatively to prevent relapse or to control hormonal hypersecretion.

• The efficacy of radiation therapy varies widely mainly depending on the type of tumor, degree of hormonal hypersecretion and radiation technique, and schedule used.

• With the advances in radiation planning and delivery, the long-term complications have improved, although hypopituitarism remains the protagonist in the list of adverse sequelae.

INTRODUCTION

Radiation therapy is widely used in the management of intracranial (including sellar and parasellar) and systemic disorders. These intracranial disorders mainly include pituitary adenomas, other (para)sellar tumors (eg, craniopharyngiomas, meningiomas, germinomas, schwannomas, chordomas/chordosarcomas, hemangiopericytomas, gliomas, pituicytomas, pinealomas, medulloblastomas, brain metastases, and vascular malformations), hematologic malignancies (eg, acute lymphoblastic leukemia, lymphomas), and face, neck, and skull base tumors (eg, nasopharyngeal carcinomas).[1] Although in many cases the irradiation aims to prevent the growth or regrowth and to control the hormonal hypersecretion of a pituitary tumor, in many others, it adversely affects the hypothalamo-pituitary function simply because this area receives significant doses of radiation offered for non–hypothalamo-pituitary disorders.

The authors have nothing to disclose.
Department of Endocrinology, Oxford Centre for Diabetes, Endocrinology and Metabolism, Churchill Hospital, Old Road, Headington, Oxford OX3 7LJ, UK
* Corresponding author.
E-mail address: niki.karavitaki@ouh.nhs.uk

Endocrinol Metab Clin N Am 44 (2015) 117–126
http://dx.doi.org/10.1016/j.ecl.2014.10.009
0889-8529/15/$ – see front matter © 2015 Elsevier Inc. All rights reserved.

This review focuses on the efficacy of various types of radiation techniques in the most common pituitary tumors and on the complications after irradiation, including in the hypothalamo-pituitary area.

EFFICACY OF PITUITARY IRRADIATION

The aim of radiation treatments to the sellar region is to prevent tumor (re)growth and to control the hormonal hypersection while sparing the surrounding normal structures. Conventional fractionated radiotherapy delivers megavoltage doses of irradiation in fractions separated over time. The irradiation is given through multiple beams from a high-energy radiation source focused on the tumor. Radiation treatments are most commonly delivered through photons (high-energy x-rays) generated by a linear accelerator (LINAC). Cobalt 60 as a source of high-energy gamma radiation has been mostly replaced, with the exception of a multiheaded cobalt unit (gamma knife). Charged particle beams in the form of photons and, more recently, helium and carbon ions have been also used as therapeutic radiation sources. Localized irradiation is achieved by offering treatment in 3 to 4 beams each shaped to conform to the shape of the tumor by using a multileaf collimator. Multileaf collimator leaves can also modulate the intensity of radiation (intensity-modulated radiotherapy [IMRT]).[1] In pituitary adenomas, the most commonly used protocol includes a total dose of 45 to 50 Gy offered in fractions of 1.6 to 1.8 Gy, 4 to 5 times per week over 5 to 6 weeks. Stereotactic techniques are related with further improvement in immobilization using relocatable or fixed frames, improved imaging, and more precise treatment delivery. Stereotactic irradiation is offered as single-fraction radiotherapy using either cobalt 60 gamma radiation emitting sources (gamma knife) or a LINAC or as stereotactic conformal radiotherapy delivered as fractionated treatment using a LINAC.

Acromegaly

The aims of the treatment of acromegaly are to inhibit growth hormone (GH) hypersecretion, normalize insulin-like growth factor-1 (IGF-1) levels and reduce or control tumor growth, leading to symptom control and minimizing the associated clinical signs and comorbidities.[2] Biochemical control is generally defined as a normal IGF-I for age and gender and a GH less than 1.0 ng/mL on an oral glucose tolerance test. With sensitive assays, a GH of less than 0.4 ng/mL would be consistent with remission.[2] Radiotherapy is generally reserved as third- or second-line treatment in cases in which surgery or medical therapy have not achieved tumor growth control or normalization of hormone levels. It may also be used for those on medical therapy aiming to stop it after the irradiation has led to hormonal control.[2] Based on series with strict remission criteria, fractionated radiotherapy achieves remission rates in 50% to 60% of the patients within 10 years (**Table 1**). Predictive factors for remission are the initial GH and IGF-I levels.[3,4] Within the first 2 years after irradiation, the GH levels are found to decrease by 50% to 70% followed by a slow gradual reduction over the next 10 to 20 years.[5] Data on the efficacy of fractionated proton beam irradiation in acromegaly are limited with no conclusive evidence on the superiority of this treatment. Stereotactic radiosurgery has been used in patients with small residual tumor, not close to the optic pathways, and biochemical remission has been reported in 35% to 100%; the variable rates reflect the different observation periods and the different criteria used to assess control of the disease.[6]

Table 1
Series with outcome of fractionated radiotherapy in patients with acromegaly

Reference	Type of Radiotherapy	No. of Patients	Follow-Up	Remission Criteria	Remission Rate (%)
Thalassinos et al,[20] 1998	Conventional	46	Mean 7.6 y	GH <2.5 ng/mL	21
Barrande et al,[3] 2000	Conventional	128	Mean 11.5 y	GH <2.5 mcg/l	53 at 10 y
Epaminonda et al,[21] 2001	Conventional	67	Mean 10 y	GH <2.5 mcg/l IGF-I normal	58 55
Jenkins et al,[4] 2006	Conventional	656	Median 7 y	GH <2.5 ng/mL IGF-I normal	60 at 10 y 63 at 10 y
Minniti et al,[22] 2006	Fractionated stereotactic	18	Median 39 mo	GH <2.5 ng/mL or GH <1 ng/mL on oral glucose tolerance test and IGF-I normal	50 at 5 y

Abbreviations: GH, growth hormone; IGF-1, insulin-like growth factor-1.
   Data from Refs.[3,4,20–22]

Cushing's Disease

Radiotherapy is almost exclusively used as a second rather than as a primary choice therapy in corticotroph adenomas after noncurative surgery (in these cases medical treatment is usually offered until irradiation provides the desired results). The most widely accepted criterion to define remission after irradiation is normalization of the 24-hour urinary free cortisol level, but additional criteria (normal basal adrenocorticotropic hormone [ACTH] or cortisol levels and suppression of cortisol on low-dose dexamethasone test) are variably used. The remission rates of hypercortisolism range from 42% to 83% without clear difference between the types of radiotherapy used (**Table 2**). Patients with Cushing's disease seem to have a shorter latency before achieving remission compared with those with acromegaly. Corticotroph tumor control is reported in 93% to 100% of the cases.[7]

Prolactinomas

Radiotherapy is reserved for patients with prolactinoma not responding to dopamine agonists or surgery or in the rare cases of malignant adenoma.[8] It aims to control tumor growth and to achieve normoprolactinemia. The hormonal response rates vary widely (0%–100%).[8]

Nonfunctioning Pituitary Adenomas

Currently, radiotherapy is offered postoperatively to patients with nonfunctioning pituitary adenomas less frequently than previously, mainly because of the long-term risk of hypopituitarism, and its indications are still not absolutely evident.[9] However, it is generally accepted that radiotherapy is not required in patients with no residual tumor, as the risk of relapse is very low.[10] Based on several series, the 5-year regrowth rate after postoperative irradiation ranges between 0% and 28%.[11–13] Randomized studies comparing surgery with or without radiotherapy are lacking; however, a report comparing the results of 2 institutions in the United Kingdom with different treatment strategies clearly showed the benefit of radiotherapy on tumor recurrence.[14] Gamma

Table 2
Series with outcome of radiotherapy in patients with Cushing's disease

Reference	Type of Radiotherapy	No. of Patients	Follow-Up	Remission Criteria	Remission Rate (%)
Nagesser et al,[23] 2000	Conventional	86	Mean 18 y	Clinical remission/normal excretion of urinary steroids/serum cortisol <80 nmol/L on low-dose dexamethasone suppression test	64
Höybye et al,[24] 2001	Gamma knife	18	Mean 17 y	Clinical remission/normal or low serum cortisol and plasma ACTH/ normal or subnormal urinary free cortisol/ normal response on dexamethasone suppression test	83
Castinetti et al,[25] 2007	Gamma knife	40	Mean 5 y	Normal urinary free cortisol/normal response on low-dose dexamethasone suppression test	42
Jagannathan et al,[26] 2007	Gamma knife	90	Mean 4 y	Normal urinary free cortisol	54
Minniti et al,[27] 2007	Conventional	40	Mean 9 y	Normal urinary free cortisol/serum cortisol/ normal response on overnight dexamethasone suppression test	78
Petit et al,[28] 2008	Proton stereotactic	33	Mean 5 y	Normal urinary free cortisol	52

Data from Refs.[23–28]

knife radiosurgery offers tumor stabilization in 60% to 78% during mean/median follow-up periods of 45 to 78 months with rates of tumor recurrence between 3% and 7%.[15]

Craniopharyngiomas

Until 1937, when Carpenter and colleagues[16] first described the beneficial effects of radiotherapy after aspiration of cyst contents in 4 cases, craniopharyngiomas were considered radioresistant.[17] The benefit of radiotherapy in preventing tumor recurrence has been shown in several reports. Series with radiologic confirmation of the radicality of resection show that the recurrence rates after gross total removal range between 0% and 62% at 10 years of follow-up. These rates are significantly lower than those reported after partial or subtotal resection (25%–100% at 10 years of follow-up). In cases of limited surgery, adjuvant radiotherapy improves significantly the local control rates (recurrence rates 10%–63% at 10 years of follow-up).[17,18] Finally, radiotherapy alone provides 10-year recurrence rates ranging between 0% and 23%.[17] These results were based on conventional fractionated external beam radiotherapy, and tumor control rates with newer higher-precision techniques, such

Table 3
Complications of pituitary irradiation

Complications	Type	Comments
Short-term	Temporary skin changes (erythema)	Resolve spontaneously within days to weeks after the completion of therapy.
	Hair loss	
	Tiredness	
	Nausea	
	Headache	
	Hearing problems	
Long-term	Radiation-induced hypopituitarism	Attributed to degenerative changes in glial cells leading to lack of trophic neural support, demyelination, and hypothalamic damage as well as to vascular derangements leading to endothelial cell death, obliteration of small vessels, and tissue necrosis.
		Onset and severity affected by total radiation dose, dose fractionation (fraction size and time between fractions for tissue repair), length of follow-up (as late as 15–20 y after irradiation) and previous damage to the hypothalamo-pituitary system (eg, compression by tumor or surgery).
		There is differential radiosensitivity with GH and gonadotroph axes being affected first, followed by ACTH and TSH axes damage (also central precocious puberty may occur with doses 18–24 Gy).
		Frequencies for each axis and dose regimes are shown in **Table 4**.
		Predictors of pituitary dysfunction after gamma knife radiosurgery include mean dose to stalk/pituitary (cutoffs 15.7 and 7.3 Gy, respectively). During median follow-up of 63 mo, new hormone deficits reported in 29% of patients after 7.6–13.2 Gy, in 39% after 13.3–19.1 Gy, and in 83% after >19.1 Gy.
		Annual long-term surveillance of the pituitary function is required.
	Radiation-induced hyperprolactinemia	Attributed to hypothalamic damage and reduction of dopamine.
		Mainly following total dose >30 Gy.
		20%–50% in adults—less common in children.
		Gradual decline may occur with time suggesting direct radiation-induced damage to lactotroph cells.
	Cranial neuropathy	Multiple cranial nerves, including II, III, IV, V, and VI, are at risk with reported rates 1.3%–0.6% after various types of radiotherapy.
	Radiation-induced optic neuropathy	Typically presents with sudden, painless, unilateral visual loss, although bilateral involvement may rapidly follow. Visual acuity decreases to a variable degree, and visual fields may show any pattern of optic nerve or chiasmal defects. No effective treatment.
		Attributed to microvascular obliteration in optic pathways.
		Onset ranges between 3 mo to >8 y after radiation exposure.
		Conventional radiotherapy may cause optic neuropathy resulting in visual deficit in 1%–3% and radiosurgery in 2%–5% of the patients.

(continued on next page)

Table 3
(continued)

Complications	Type	Comments
		Susceptibility increases with increasing age, comorbid diabetes, preexisting compression to the optic nerves and chiasm, volume of the optic apparatus exposed to high-dose irradiation (for gamma knife), and prior external beam radiation therapy.
		Frequency is dose dependent, increasing with total doses >50–55 Gy (fractionated radiotherapy) or single doses >10 Gy (stereotactic radiosurgery) or radiation fraction size >2 Gy (fractionated radiotherapy) or total dose to the optic pathway >8 Gy. For tumors close to the chiasm, even total doses of 45 Gy may cause optic neuropathy, and the distance between tumor margin and optic apparatus should be at least 3 mm.
	Radiation-induced brain necrosis	May occur in the treated peritumoral area or distal from the original tumor but always within the radiation fields. The patients may present with raised intracranial pressure because of edema, cognitive dysfunction, seizures or focal neurologic signs related to the position of the lesion.
		Related with microvascular obliteration, ischemic necrosis, and demyelination of white matter.
		Onset ranges between a few months to >40 y after the irradiation.
		The risk increases with increasing total dose and fraction size and it is almost unknown with total doses 45–50 Gy in fractions of <2 Gy.
	Cerebrovascular accidents	Cerebrovascular mortality has been found increased in patients with pituitary adenoma treated by radiotherapy compared with the general population.
		Related to atherogenesis to the vascular lining from the radiotoxicity.
		Risk factors include older age, previous aggressive intracranial surgery and total dose >45 Gy.
		Particularly in patients with acromegaly, radiotherapy has been associated with increased mortality with cerebrovascular disease being the main cause of death.
	Second brain tumor	In a series of patients irradiated for pituitary adenoma probability 2% at 20 y, but another series comparing patients with pituitary adenoma and treated by surgery alone or postoperative radiotherapy did not confirm increased risk.
		Most commonly meningiomas, gliomas, chondrosarcomas.
		Risk factors including radiation thresholds not defined.
	Cognitive dysfunction	No consistent data and in studies using extensive psychometric testing the effect of irradiation could not be clearly distinguished from that of other interventions or of the tumor itself.
	Quality of life	Patients with nonfunctioning pituitary adenoma treated by radiotherapy show compromised scores in the areas of energy levels and perception of the overall health in health-related quality-of-life questionnaires.

Abbreviations: ACTH, adrenocorticotropic hormone; TSH, thyroid-stimulating hormone.
Data from Refs.[120,41]

as fractionated stereotactic conformal radiotherapy, have remained optimal with 5-year progression-free survival more than 90%.[19] The beneficial effect of radio-therapy (regardless of whether preceded by second surgery) in recurrent lesions has been clearly shown.[18] Stereotactic radiosurgery achieves tumor control in a substantial number of patients with small-volume lesions, and reported 5-year progression-free survival rates range between 61% and 68%.[19] This treatment may be particularly useful for well-defined residual disease after surgery or for the treatment of small solid recurrent tumors, particularly after failure of conventional radiotherapy.

COMPLICATIONS OF PITUITARY IRRADIATION

These are shown in **Tables 3** and **4** with the most common being radiation-induced hypopituitarism.

FUTURE CONSIDERATIONS

Irradiation remains an important tool in our therapeutic armamentarium for intracranial (including sellar and parasellar) and systemic disorders. Studies comparing the efficacy and safety of different radiation techniques—particularly for sellar and parasellar lesions—are required, aiming to provide reliable data on the place of each technique in the management algorithm. Furthermore, prospective studies of consecutive,

Table 4
Hypopituitarism after cranial radiotherapy

Condition Treated with Radiotherapy	Radiation Details	Pituitary Hormone Deficits
Leukemia and lymphoma	Fractionated total body irradiation (7–16 Gy)	Isolated GH deficiency in children
Leukemia and lymphoma	Fractionated prophylactic cranial irradiation (18–24 Gy)	GH deficiency in children Small risk of other deficits in children/adults
Nonpituitary brain tumors	Conventional fractionated cranial irradiation (30–50 Gy)	GH deficiency 30%–100% (higher in children) FSH/LH deficiency ~30% ACTH deficiency ~20%–30% TSH deficiency ~10%
Nasopharyngeal carcinoma and skull-base tumors	Conventional fractionated cranial irradiation (50–70 Gy)	GH deficiency 55%–100% FSH/LH deficiency ~35%–82% ACTH deficiency ~18%–25% TSH deficiency ~15%–45%
Pituitary tumors	Conventional fractionated cranial irradiation (30–50 Gy)	GH deficiency ~100% FSH/LH deficiency ~65% ACTH deficiency ~40%–50% TSH deficiency ~50%

Limitations of the studies these data rely on include selection bias of patients (eg, only the symptomatic ones may have been tested), various sample sizes, different diagnostic tests and criteria, various radiotherapy schedules (biological effective dose not usually estimated), variable follow-up, impact of previous cranial surgery, or chemotherapy.

Abbreviations: ACTH, adrenocorticotropic hormone; FSH, follicle-stimulating hormone; GH, growth hormone; LH, luteinizing hormone; TSH, thyroid-stimulating hormone.
Data from Refs.[1,33,42,43]

nonselected patients relying on robust diagnostic criteria and on the biological effective dose to the hypothalamus-pituitary are needed to clarify timing and frequency of damage to each axis and to provide the basis for safe and cost-effective surveillance protocols.

REFERENCES

1. Fernadez A, Brada M, Zabulliene L, et al. Radiation-induced hypopituitarism. Endocr Relat Cancer 2009;16:733–72.
2. Melmed S, Colao A, Barkan A, et al. Guidelines for acromegaly management: an update. J Clin Endocrinol Metab 2009;94:1509–17.
3. Barrande G, Pittino-Lungo M, Coste J, et al. Hormonal and metabolic effects of radiotherapy in acromegaly: long-term results in 128 patients followed in a single center. J Clin Endocrinol Metab 2000;85:3779–85.
4. Jenkins PJ, Bates P, Carson MN, et al. Conventional pituitary irradiation is effective in lowering serum growth hormone and insulin-like growth factor-I in patients with acromegaly. J Clin Endocrinol Metab 2006;91:1239–45.
5. Castinetti F, Morange I, Dufour H, et al. Radiotherapy and radiosurgery in acromegaly. Pituitary 2009;12:3–10.
6. Minniti G, Scaringi C, Enrici M. Radiation techniques for acromegaly. Radiat Oncol 2011;6:167–74.
7. Losa M, Picozzi P, Redaelli MG, et al. Pituitary radiotherapy for Cushing's disease. Neuroendocrinology 2010;92(Suppl 1):107–10.
8. Sheplan Olsen LJ, Robles Irizarry L, Chao ST, et al. Radiotherapy for prolactin-secreting pituitary tumors. Pituitary 2012;15:135–45.
9. Wass JA, Reddy R, Karavitaki N. The post-operative monitoring of non-functioning pituitary adenomas. Nat Rev Endocrinol 2011;7:431–4.
10. Reddy R, Cudlip S, Byrne RV, et al. Can we ever stop imaging in surgically treated and radiotherapy naïve patients with non-functioning pituitary adenoma? Eur J Endocrinol 2011;165:739–44.
11. Woollons AC, Hunn MK, Rajapakse YR, et al. Non-functioning pituitary adenomas: indications for postoperative radiotherapy. Clin Endocrinol (Oxf) 2000;53:713–7.
12. Park P, Chandler WF, Barkan A, et al. The role of radiation therapy after surgical resection of non-functional pituitary adenomas. Neurosurgery 2004;55:100–7.
13. Dekkers OM, Pereira AM, Roelfsema F, et al. Observation alone after transsphenoidal surgery for non-functioning pituitary macroadenoma. J Clin Endocrinol Metab 2006;91:1796–801.
14. Gittoes NJ, Bates AS, Tse W, et al. Radiotherapy for non-functioning pituitary tumours. Clin Endocrinol (Oxf) 1998;48:331–7.
15. Castinetti F, Régis J, Dufour H, et al. Role of stereotactic radiosurgery in the management of pituitary adenomas. Nat Rev Endocrinol 2010;6:214–23.
16. Carpenter RC, Chamberlin GW, Frazier CH, et al. The treatment of hypophyseal stalk tumours by evacuation and irradiation. Am J Roentgenol 1937;38:162–7.
17. Karavitaki N, Cudlip S, Adams CB, et al. Craniopharyngiomas. Endocr Rev 2006; 27:371–97.
18. Karavitaki N, Brufani C, Warner JT, et al. Craniopharyngiomas in children and adults: systematic analysis of 121 cases with long-term follow-up. Clin Endocrinol (Oxf) 2005;62:397–409.
19. Karavitaki N. Management of craniopharyngiomas. J Endocrinol Invest 2014;37: 219–20.

20. Thalassinos NC, Tsagarakis S, Ioannides G, et al. Megavoltage pituitary irradiation lowers but seldom leads to safe GH levels in acromegaly: a long-term follow-up study. Eur J Endocrinol 1998;138:160–3.
21. Epaminonda P, Porretti S, Cappiello V, et al. Efficacy of radiotherapy in normalising serum IGF-I, acid-labile subunit (ALS) and IGFBP-3 levels in acromegaly. Clin Endocrinol (Oxf) 2001;55:183–9.
22. Minniti G, Traish D, Ashley S, et al. Fractionated stereotactic conformal radiotherapy for secreting and nonsecreting pituitary adenomas. Clin Endocrinol (Oxf) 2006;64:542–8.
23. Nagesser SK, van Seters AP, Kievit J, et al. Treatment of pituitary-dependent Cushing's syndrome: long-term results of unilateral adrenalectomy followed by external pituitary irradiation compared to transsphenoidal pituitary surgery. Clin Endocrinol (Oxf) 2000;52:427–35.
24. Höybye C, Grenbäck E, Rähn T, et al. Adrenocorticotropic hormone-producing pituitary tumors: 12- to 22-year follow-up after treatment with stereotactic radiosurgery. Neurosurgery 2001;49:284–91 [discussion: 291–2].
25. Castinetti F, Nagai M, Dufour H, et al. Gamma knife radiosurgery is a successful adjunctive treatment in Cushing's disease. Eur J Endocrinol 2007;156:91–8.
26. Jagannathan J, Sheehan JP, Pouratian N, et al. Gamma Knife surgery for Cushing's disease. J Neurosurg 2007;106:980–7.
27. Minniti G, Osti M, Jaffrain-Rea ML, et al. Long-term follow-up results of postoperative radiation therapy for Cushing's disease. J Neurooncol 2007;84:79–84.
28. Petit JH, Biller BM, Yock TI, et al. Proton stereotactic radiotherapy for persistent adrenocorticotropin-producing adenomas. J Clin Endocrinol Metab 2008;93: 393–9.
29. Constine LS, Woolf PD, Cann D, et al. Hypothalamic-pituitary dysfunction after radiation for brain tumors. N Engl J Med 1993;328:87–94.
30. Brada M, Rajan B, Traish D, et al. The long-term efficacy of conservative surgery and radiotherapy in the control of pituitary adenomas. Clin Endocrinol (Oxf) 1993; 38:571–8.
31. Tishler RB, Loeffler JS, Lunsford LD, et al. Tolerance of cranial nerves of the cavernous sinus to radiosurgery. Int J Radiat Oncol Biol Phys 1993;27:215–21.
32. Brada M, Ashley S, Ford D, et al. Cerebrovascular mortality in patients with pituitary adenoma. Clin Endocrinol (Oxf) 2002;57:713–7.
33. Darzy KH, Shalet SM. Hypopituitarism following radiotherapy. Pituitary 2009;12: 40–50.
34. Leenstra JL, Tanaka S, Kline RW, et al. Factors associated with endocrine deficits after stereotactic radiosurgery of pituitary adenomas. Neurosurgery 2010;67: 27–32.
35. Sattler MG, van Beek AP, Wolffenbuttel BH, et al. The incidence of second tumours and mortality in pituitary adenoma patients treated with postoperative radiotherapy versus surgery alone. Radiother Oncol 2012;104:125–30.
36. Sicignano G, Losa M, del Vecchio A, et al. Dosimetric factors associated with pituitary function after Gamma Knife Surgery (GKS) of pituitary adenomas. Radiother Oncol 2012;104:119–24.
37. Sheehan JP, Starke RM, Mathieu D, et al. Gamma Knife radiosurgery for the management of nonfunctioning pituitary adenomas: a multicenter study. J Neurosurg 2013;119:446–56.
38. Leavitt JA, Stafford SL, Link MJ, et al. Long-term evaluation of radiation-induced optic neuropathy after single-fraction stereotactic radiosurgery. Int J Radiat Oncol Biol Phys 2013;87:524–7.

39. Capatina C, Christodoulides C, Fernandez A, et al. Current treatment protocols can offer a normal or near-normal quality of life in the majority of patients with non-functioning pituitary adenomas. Clin Endocrinol (Oxf) 2013;78:86–93.

40. Ayuk J, Clayton RN, Holder G, et al. Growth hormone and pituitary radiotherapy, but not serum insulin-like growth factor-I concentrations, predict excess mortality in patients with acromegaly. J Clin Endocrinol Metab 2004;89:1613–7.

41. Mestron A, Webb SM, Astorga R, et al. Epidemiology, clinical characteristics, outcome, morbidity and mortality in acromegaly based on the Spanish Acromegaly registry (Registro Espanol de Acromegalia, REA). Eur J Endocrinol 2004;151:439–46.

42. Agha A, Sherlock M, Brennan S, et al. Hypothalamic-pituitary dysfunction after irradiation of nonpituitary brain tumors in adults. J Clin Endocrinol Metab 2005; 90:6355–60.

43. Appelman-Dijkstra NM, Kokshoorn NE, Dekkers OM, et al. Pituitary dysfunction in adult patients after cranial radiotherapy: systematic review and meta-analysis. J Clin Endocrinol Metab 2011;96:2330–40.

Hypopituitarism
Growth Hormone and Corticotropin Deficiency

Cristina Capatina, MD[a,b], John A.H. Wass, MD, FRCP[c,d],*

KEYWORDS

- Hypopituitarism • Growth hormone • Adults • Corticotropin • ACTH • Deficiency
- Replacement treatment

KEY POINTS

- Adult growth hormone deficiency (AGHD) is associated with increased cardiovascular risk and alterations in substrate metabolism, in addition to impaired body composition, muscle strength, bone mass, and quality of life.
- Growth hormone (GH) replacement therapy with individualized dosing regimens improves most features of the clinical syndrome of AGHD.
- Corticotropin deficiency (central adrenal insufficiency; CAI) can present with chronic, nonspecific symptoms, or acutely, with life-threatening adrenal crisis.
- If acute CAI is suspected, immediate treatment should be initiated.
- Chronic management of CAI requires lifelong glucocorticoid administration with mandatory dose adjustment during stressful events.

INTRODUCTION

Hypopituitarism refers to the decreased secretion of 1 or more pituitary hormones caused by pituitary or hypothalamic disease. The clinical manifestations of hypopituitarism depend on its cause, in addition to the type and severity of the hormonal deficit. In most etiologic scenarios, the secretion of gonadotropins and growth hormone (GH) are more likely to be affected than corticotropin (adrenocorticotropic hormone; ACTH) and thyroid-stimulating hormone (TSH), but isolated deficiencies of any hormone can

The authors have nothing to disclose.
[a] Department of Endocrinology, C.I. Parhon National Institute of Endocrinology, Carol Davila University of Medicine and Pharmacy, 34-36 Aviatorilor Boulevard, Bucharest 011863, Romania; [b] Department of Pituitary and Neuroendocrine Diseases, C.I. Parhon National Institute of Endocrinology, 34-36 Aviatorilor Boulevard, Bucharest 011863, Romania; [c] Discipline of Endocrinology and Diabetes, University of Oxford, Old Road, Headington, Oxford OX3 7LE, UK; [d] Department of Endocrinology, Oxford Centre for Diabetes, Endocrinology and Metabolism, Churchill Hospital, Old Road, Headington, Oxford OX3 7LE, UK
* Corresponding author. Department of Endocrinology, Oxford Centre for Diabetes, Endocrinology and Metabolism, Churchill Hospital, Old Road, Headington, Oxford OX3 7LE, UK.
E-mail address: john.wass@noc.anglox.nhs.uk

Endocrinol Metab Clin N Am 44 (2015) 127–141
http://dx.doi.org/10.1016/j.ecl.2014.11.002
0889-8529/15/$ – see front matter © 2015 Elsevier Inc. All rights reserved.

occur. The diagnosis is made by separately documenting the subnormal secretion of each pituitary hormone. The treatment of ACTH deficiency (central adrenal insufficiency; CAI) is life saving and consists of lifelong glucocorticoid administration. The treatment of adult growth hormone deficiency (AGHD) consists of recombinant human GH (rhGH) preparations according to criteria devised by national regulatory bodies.

ETIOLOGY

In most cases of acquired AGHD and CAI, the etiology is common with that of other types of noninherited hypopituitarism (**Box 1**).[1,2] Most frequently, a pituitary adenoma

---

Box 1
Etiology of growth hormone (GH) and corticotropin (ACTH) deficiency in adults

Acquired Causes of Adult Growth Hormone Deficiency and/or Adult Central Adrenal Insufficiency (CAI)

- Pituitary tumor
- Craniopharyngioma
- Pituitary/brain surgery
- Pituitary/brain irradiation
- Other central nervous system tumor, including metastatic tumor in the hypothalamic/pituitary area
- Traumatic brain injury
- Subarachnoid hemorrhage
- Empty sella syndrome
- Granulomatous diseases (hemochromatosis, sarcoidosis, Wegener granulomatosis, histiocytosis)
- Infectious diseases (tuberculosis, actinomycosis)
- Hypophysitis (can cause isolated CAI)
- Pituitary apoplexy
- Internal carotid artery aneurism

For CAI only: adult-onset isolated CAI (mostly autoimmune, frequently as part of polyglandular autoimmune syndrome); drug-induced (exogenous glucocorticoids, mifepristone, various antipsychotics); following total removal of an ACTH-secreting pituitary adenoma

Congenital Causes of Growth Hormone Deficiency (GHD) and CAI

GHD

- Isolated
- Combined pituitary deficiencies:
  - Mutations of *PROP1, HESX1, LHX3, LHX4, POU1F1* (encoding PIT1)
  - Associated with brain structural defects

CAI

- Isolated congenital CAI (*POMC* or *TPIT* gene mutations, POMC processing defect)
- Combined pituitary deficiencies:
  - Mutations of *PROP1, HESX1, LHX3, LHX4* (panhypopituitarism)
  - Midline forebrain defects

or craniopharyngioma, or their treatment, are responsible, and multiple pituitary deficiencies are present.

Some childhood-onset cases of GH deficiency (GHD), resulting from well-defined congenital conditions, account for almost a quarter of AGHD cases; by contrast, idiopathic childhood-onset GHD frequently disappears in adulthood.[3] Idiopathic isolated adult-onset GHD[4] or CAI[1] have been rarely described, an autoimmune cause being suspected in many cases.[1]

ADULT GROWTH HORMONE DEFICIENCY
Epidemiology

The incidence of AGHD has been estimated at 1 in every 100,000 persons per year[5] and the prevalence in the general population about 27.75 per 100.000, more frequently in tumoral etiology.[6]

Health Effects of Adult Growth Hormone Deficiency and Benefits of Growth Hormone Replacement

AGHD has been associated with adverse changes in body composition,[7] muscle strength,[8] quality of life (QoL),[9] cardiovascular risk factors,[10] bone mass,[11] and possible reduced life expectancy (**Table 1**).[12]

Table 1
Summary of the main findings in AGHD and the response to GH treatment

Untreated GHD	GH Replacement Effect	Comments
Adverse body composition[7] ↑ BF ↓ LBM ↑ WHR	Reversal of adverse changes[13] ↓ BF (mainly visceral) ↑ LBM (mainly proximal) ↓ WHR	Effect on BF not sustained long term[13]
↓ Skeletal muscle mass and strength[8]	Slow, progressive ↑ in muscle mass and force[8]	
↓ BMD[11] ↑ Fracture rate[14]	Initial ↑ (for a few years) then preservation of bone mass[15] Limited data on fractures rate	
Dyslipidemia[21] ↑ Total LDL cholesterol ↓ HDL cholesterol ↑ Triglycerides	Reversal[22] ↓ Total LDL cholesterol No effect on triglycerides; variable on HDL cholesterol	Effect of treatment in both short-term and long-term administration[22]
Proinflammatory status (↑ IL-6, CRP)[23] Premature atherosclerosis[25] ↑ IMT ↑ Atheromatous plaques ↑ Arterial stiffness	↓ Inflammation markers[24] Slow reversal of atherosclerotic changes with long-term treatment[26]	Possibly contributing to decreasing CV risk during GH treatment
Insulin resistance[19]	Controversial long-term effects[20]	
Decreased QoL and well being[9]	Progressive improvement in affected QoL areas[9]	Preferably monitored with specific questionnaires (AGHDA)

Abbreviations: ↑, increase; ↓, decrease; AGHDA, Assessment of Growth Hormone Deficiency in Adults; BF, body fat; BMD, bone mineral density; CRP, C-reactive protein; CV, cardiovascular; GH, growth hormone; GHD, growth hormone deficiency; HDL, high-density lipoprotein; IL, interleukin; IMT, intima-media thickness; LBM, lean body mass; LDL, low-density lipoprotein; QoL, quality of life; WHR, waist-to-hip ratio.

Body composition
The body composition in AGHD recognizes changes known to be associated with increased cardiovascular risk. The ability of GH replacement to partially reverse these changes is well documented. Long-term replacement induces sustained effects on lean body mass but not on body fat.[13]

Muscle strength and exercise performance
Untreated AGHD patients have reduced isometric muscle strength and mass, and significant long-term treatment benefits have been described.[8]

Bone health
AGHD patients have decreased bone mineral density (BMD) in comparison with normal individuals.[11] Consequently, their fracture risk is also increased (almost 3 times compared with controls), especially in men.[14]

Long-term BMD increases have been reported, mostly for the first 5 years, followed by preservation of bone mass.[15] Data regarding the effect on fractures are limited; rhGH treatment decreased the rate of radiologic vertebral fractures in one study.[16]

Mortality and cardiovascular effects
In hypopituitary patients not receiving GH replacement, an increased standardized mortality ratio has been described, attributed mainly to vascular causes.[12] However, only very few cases had been formally tested for GHD in this study, and GHD was not confirmed as an independent predictor for increased mortality. By contrast, treated AGHD patients in the KIMS database have mortality similar to that of the normal population.[17]

The evidence for the etiologic connection between AGHD and adverse cardiovascular effects is notably stronger. An increased rate of cardiovascular and cerebrovascular events was demonstrated in untreated AGHD patients.[18] The association is multifactorial: various cardiovascular risk factors (proinflammatory status, atherosclerotic changes, adverse lipid profile) are associated with AGHD and are reversed by rhGH treatment (see **Table 1**).

Insulin sensitivity is decreased in AGHD patients in comparison with controls.[19] The overall effect during treatment, however, is controversial. A meta-analysis including both short-term and long-term studies demonstrated an overall increase in both fasting glucose and insulin.[20]

Quality of life
Another major characteristic of GHD is impaired QoL, particularly related to the energy level, emotional reaction, and general and mental health,[9] ideally assessed with specifically designed standardized questionnaires such as the AGHDA (Assessment of Growth Hormone Deficiency in Adults). Sustained long-term improvement with treatment has been demonstrated.[9]

Diagnosis

Testing for AGHD is recommended in specific subgroups of patients (**Box 2**).

Serum measurement of insulin-like growth factor (IGF)-I has low diagnostic sensitivity: significant overlap between AGHD patients and healthy subjects occurs, especially in the elderly.[27] However, very low IGF-I levels have 95% diagnostic accuracy,[28] especially in hypopituitary patients.[27] In these patients provocative testing is not mandatory,[27] but must be performed in all the others (**Table 2**).

The evaluation of spontaneous GH secretion over 24 hours or IGF-binding protein 3 is inappropriate as a diagnostic test for AGHD.[29]

Box 2
Indications for GHD testing

- Signs and symptoms of hypothalamic or pituitary disease
- After cranial irradiation or surgery in the hypothalamus/pituitary area: repeated testing after radiotherapy
- Twelve months after traumatic brain injury (TBI) or subarachnoid hemorrhage (SAH)

In all these cases, an intention to treat should be present before testing.

- Retesting of childhood-onset GHD after completion of growth (except cases with specific proven mutations, structural congenital defects, irreversible hypothalamic-pituitary damage)

Data from Cook DM, Yuen KC, Biller BM, et al. American Association of Clinical Endocrinologists medical guidelines for clinical practice for growth hormone use in growth hormone-deficient adults and transition patients—2009 update. Endocr Pract 2009;Suppl 15:21–9; and Ho KK. Consensus guidelines for the diagnosis and treatment of adults with GH deficiency II: a statement of the GH Research Society in association with the European Society for Pediatric Endocrinology, Lawson Wilkins Society, European Society of Endocrinology, Japan Endocrine Society, and Endocrine Society of Australia. Eur J Endocrinol 2007;157(6):695–700.

Stimulation tests recommended by the consensus guidelines are the insulin tolerance test (ITT), growth hormone–releasing hormone (GHRH) + arginine, GHRH + growth hormone–releasing peptide, and glucagon tests,[30,31] all used to variable degree in Europe and the United States.

The somatotropic response to all agents is blunted in obese patients, sometimes overlapping with that of hypopituitary patients.[32] Appropriate weight-based cutoffs are needed to avoid false-positive diagnoses in these cases.

Treatment

Evidence supporting the beneficial effects of rhGH replacement in AGHD led to the widespread approval of rhGH treatment in AGHD. All patients with severe AGHD are eligible for GH replacement. In some countries, such as the United Kingdom, significant QoL impairment must be additionally present.

Dosing

Initially a body-weight–based dosing regimen was used, leading to higher doses and increased incidence of adverse effects (mostly fluid retention). At present, individualized titration dosing based on IGF-I levels is recommended,[31] achieving lower daily GH doses with similar benefits and fewer side effects.[37]

As GH secretion is increased in the young and in women, the recommended starting dose is differentiated (**Box 3**).[30,31]

Monitoring

Clinical, anthropometric, and cardiovascular assessment is needed during treatment (**Box 4**).[30,31]

Safety Issues

Diabetes mellitus
Mild and often transient changes in glucose metabolism occur during GH replacement in AGHD patients.[38] However, no evidence for overall increased incidence of diabetes

Table 2
Diagnostic tests for AGHD

	Test Protocol	Test Interpretation	Advantages	Disadvantages
Basal Determinations				
IGF-I	Single serum measurement	Normal value does not exclude diagnosis[31] Very low value in hypopituitary patients = GHD[27]	Screening test Most useful in hypopituitary patients	Significant overlap with normal individuals[27]
Provocative Tests (Only 1 Needed[31])				
ITT	0.1–0.15 IU/kg regular insulin IV Measure glucose, GH, and cortisol at 0, 30, 60 min Glycemia <40 mg/dL (2.2 mml/L) required for validity	3 µg/L	Simultaneous assessment of the ACTH reserve Gold standard	Contraindicated in: >60 y old Ischemic heart disease History of seizures Risk of adverse effects; requires continuous presence of a physician
Glucagon test	1–1.5 mg glucagon IM Measure glucose, GH, cortisol at 0 min and every 30 min for 4 h	3 µg/L[33]	Good diagnostic accuracy Less severe side effects	Late hypoglycemia possible[33]
GHRH–arginine	1 µg/kg GHRH bolus + 0.5 g/kg arginine IV in 30 min Measure GH at 0 min and every 30 min for 2 h	BMI-dependent[34]	Good accuracy and tolerability	GHRH unavailable in most settings
GHRH–GHRP-2	1 µg/kg GHRH + 100 µg GHRP-2 intravenously Sample for GH at baseline and every 30 min for 2 h	9 µg/L (proposed)[35] No normative data available		Decreased response in obese and elderly[35] GHRH unavailable in most settings
GHRH–GHRP-6	1 µg/kg GHRH + 1 µg/kg GHRP-6 intravenously Sample for GH at baseline and every 30 min for 2 h	10 µg/L[36]	Good accuracy and tolerability Not affected by age[36]	Decreased response in obese GHRH unavailable in most settings

Abbreviations: ACTH, corticotropin; AGHD, adult growth hormone deficiency; BMI, body mass index; GH, growth hormone; GHRH, growth hormone–releasing hormone; GHRP, growth hormone–releasing peptide; IGF-I, insulin-like growth factor I; IM, intramuscular; ITT, insulin tolerance test; IV, intravenous.

Box 3
Recommendations for GH replacement treatment

- Check the hypothalamic-pituitary-adrenal axis and replace if necessary
- Start with low doses:
  - 0.2 to 0.3 mg/d by subcutaneous injections
  - 0.1 mg/d in the elderly
- Monitor clinically and with insulin-like growth factor I (IGF-I) (frequently at the initiation of treatment)
- Increase the dose gradually, by no more than 0.1 to 0.2 mg/d, no earlier than 1 month from the previous dose change
- Aim for IGF-I in the upper half of the reference range for age and gender
- Do not choose or adjust the GH dose based on body weight

Comments:

Women on oral estrogen replacement may require higher doses

If possible, a nonoral route of estrogen administration should be preferred[31]

---

mellitus was noted[39] except in patients with other risk factors,[40] for whom careful, continuous monitoring is particularly important.

Malignancy

No increased malignancy rates[41] or malignancy-related mortality[42] were demonstrated in more recent studies.

Tumor regrowth or recurrence

There is no evidence that GH replacement in adults increases the risk of tumor regrowth or recurrence of pituitary tumors,[43] parasellar tumors,[44] or craniopharyngiomas.[45]

Concluding Remarks

GH therapy is beneficial for most patients with AGHD and, although some long-term issues still remain insufficiently clarified, current evidence does not raise significant safety concerns.

Box 4
Monitoring of recombinant human GH replacement treatment

- Careful history, paying special attention to energy, vitality, exercise performance, adverse effects
- Anthropometric (or dual x-ray absorptiometry [DXA]) measurements of the body composition, yearly
- Objective determination of quality of life, yearly
- Cardiovascular risk markers (at least serum lipids, blood pressure, electrocardiogram), yearly
- Fasting glucose, hemoglobin A_{1c}, every 6 to 12 months
- DXA osteodensitometry every 2 years
- IGF-I measurement (every 1 to 2 months at the initiation of treatment)
- When maintenance dose is reached, monitor once or twice every year
- Aim for normal age-specific and gender-specific values

CORTICOTROPIN DEFICIENCY (CENTRAL ADRENAL INSUFFICIENCY)
Epidemiology

Endogenous CAI has an estimated prevalence of 28 in 100,000,[6] much less than that of iatrogenic CAI induced by the chronic administration of glucocorticoids (not detailed in this article).

Clinical Manifestations

The clinical presentation of CAI partly overlaps with that of primary adrenal insufficiency (**Box 5**).[1,46] Signs of mineralocorticoid deficiency (severe dehydration, salt craving, hyperkalemia) are not present, as the mineralocorticoid secretion is preserved. Hyponatremia can, however, occur secondary to either inappropriate secretion of antidiuretic hormone resulting from glucocorticoid deficiency or associated central hypothyroidism.[1] Skin hyperpigmentation is absent. Symptoms and signs of the primary underlying disorder can be present.

Acute adrenal insufficiency is a life-threatening emergency presenting with severe hypotension (sometimes hypovolemic shock), vomiting, and possible acute abdominal pain or fever mimicking acute abdominal emergencies.[2] It occurs abruptly (eg, pituitary apoplexy) or during intercurrent stress in previously undiagnosed patients or those who fail to properly adapt to replacement doses.

Diagnosis

Morning serum cortisol is initially assessed, but is diagnostic only if values are extremely low (<100 nmol/L strongly suggest adrenal insufficiency)[47] or high-normal

---

Box 5
Presenting features of CAI

Symptoms and Signs

- Fatigue
- Anorexia
- Weight loss
- Nausea, vomiting
- Muscle and joint pain
- Dizziness
- Arterial hypotension (initially postural, later occurring also in clinostatism)
- Loss of axillary and pubic hair in women
- Pallor
- Fever
- Abdominal pain
- Possibly symptoms of other pituitary deficiencies

Biochemical Findings

- Hyponatremia
- Blood count abnormalities (anemia, lymphocytosis, eosinophilia)
- Hypoglycemia (rare, mostly if concurrent GH deficiency)
- Hypercalcemia

(>19 µg/dL or 500 nmol/L virtually excludes the diagnosis[48]). For intermediate values of serum cortisol, dynamic testing is required (**Table 3**).

Plasma ACTH concentration (low or low-normal in CAI) is not helpful in the initial diagnostic workup.[49]

The ITT is considered the gold standard for the evaluation of the hypothalamo-pituitary-adrenal axis.[50]

The metyrapone test shows good concordance with the ITT,[51] but its use is limited by the low availability of the compound. Close medical surveillance is needed, as both ITT and metyrapone may precipitate an acute adrenal crisis.

High-dose ACTH stimulation test (short synacthen test; SST) (250 µg synthetic $ACTH_{1-24}$) directly assesses the adrenal secretory reserve. It may not detect recent-onset or mild forms of CAI[52] so ITT may be necessary,[53] as well as in highly suspicious negative SST cases.[1,54] However, the overall concordance between SST and ITT is good,[54] and SST can be used in most cases.

The low-dose ACTH stimulation test (same as above but using 1 µg synthetic $ACTH_{1-24}$) has been described as a more sensitive diagnostic test with better concordance with ITT results.[55] However, owing to the lack of 1-µg ACTH vials and technical problems, it still has a more limited role than the standard test.

The corticotropin-releasing hormone (CRH) test has been used to differentiate hypothalamic from pituitary disease in CAI. The lack of studies involving large numbers of patients and the high cost of CRH has greatly limited the use of this test.[1]

All of these tests use serum cortisol cutoffs that can be inappropriate in conditions altering the cortisol-binding globulin status (eg, contraceptive pill use, cirrhosis, nephrotic syndrome). The use of salivary cortisol would overcome this, but validated cutoffs are lacking.

Treatment

Long-term chronic treatment

Treatment requires lifelong administration of glucocorticoids (**Box 6**). Mineralocorticoid administration is not necessary. In mild, oligosymptomatic cases, replacement therapy is only required during stressful situations.

Thrice-daily regimens more closely mimic the physiologic steroid circadian profile, and lead more frequently to optimal biochemical replacement[57] and improved QoL.[58] Supraphysiologic doses are associated with substantial morbidity.[2]

Long-acting glucocorticoids can also be used in equivalent doses, but their use may result in unfavorably high nocturnal cortisol levels.[1]

Addition of dehydroepiandrosterone (DHEA) to glucocorticoid replacement therapy may exert positive effects on well-being, mood, and sexuality in women with CAI.[59] However, its use is still controversial, mostly because of the lack of large, placebo-controlled, randomized studies and of adequate widely available preparations. A daily oral dose of DHEA sulfate, 25 to 50 mg, can be used in selected patients with decreased well-being despite glucocorticoid treatment.[60]

Morning plasma ACTH, plasma levels, and urinary cortisol levels have been proposed as tools for monitoring but, as none is fully reliable, clinical judgment has priority.

Stressful events (trauma, surgery, fever, illnesses) need special management (see **Box 6**).[2]

There is stringent need for more physiologic replacement strategies; recently approved dual-release preparations show promise,[61] but larger studies are warranted.

Acute crisis treatment

The management of acute adrenal crisis[2] is detailed in **Box 6**.

Table 3
Diagnostic tests for CAI

	Test Protocol	Test Interpretation	Advantages	Disadvantages
Basal Determinations				
Morning cortisol	8 AM fasting sampling for cortisol and ACTH	Strongly suggest diagnosis if <100 nmol/L	Easy to perform	Cannot establish the positive diagnosis
ACTH		Low-normal or normal ACTH with low cortisol suggests CAI		Careful sample processing needed Limited reliability for low values
Dynamic Tests				
ITT	0.1–0.15 IU/kg IV regular insulin Measure glucose, GH, and cortisol at 0, 30, 60 min Glycemia <40 mg/dL (2.2 mmol/L) required for a valid test	Normal response cortisol >500 nmol/L	Simultaneous assessment of the ACTH reserve	Contraindicated in: >60 y old Ischemic heart disease History of seizures Risk of adverse effects Continuous monitoring needed Can precipitate adrenal crisis
Metyrapone test	Metyrapone 30 mg/kg orally at midnight Measure cortisol, 11DOC, ACTH at 8 AM the following morning)	Cortisol + 11DOC >450 nmol/L (16.5 μg/dL)[48] ACTH 11DOC >200 nmol/L required for a valid test	Good diagnostic accuracy	Limited availability of metyrapone and 11DOC assay Can precipitate adrenal crisis Close monitoring required
Standard-dose corticotropin test	250 μg ACTH$_{1-24}$ IM or IV Measure serum cortisol at 0, 30, 60 min	Normal peak cortisol >500 nmol/L Local reference ranges recommended[56]	Good accuracy and tolerability Safe, quick test Can be performed any time of the day Good concordance with ITT	False negative in recent-onset (eg, the first weeks after pituitary surgery) or mild CAI
Low-dose corticotropin test	1 μg ACTH$_{1-24}$ IM or IV Measure serum cortisol at 0, 30, 60 min	Normal peak cortisol >500 nmol/L		Technical difficulties (dilution needed)
CRH test	1 μg/kg CRH as IV bolus Measure cortisol every 15 min for 90 min	Peak cortisol >500 nmol/L	Differentiates pituitary (blunted ACTH response) from hypothalamic disease (prolonged/exaggerated response)	Low availability High cost Less standardized

Abbreviations: CRH, corticotropin-releasing hormone; 11DOC, 11-deoxycortisol.

Box 6
Treatment of CAI

Chronic Replacement Treatment
- Hydrocortisone[a] 15 to 25 mg/d in 2 or, better, 3 doses
- Give half to two-thirds of the dose in the morning
- Medical identification bracelet or card available at all times
- Inform patients about disease, treatment, stress management
- Regularly check body weight, blood pressure, serum electrolytes
- Careful regular anamnesis looking for clinical signs of underreplacement or overreplacement

Increase Doses In:
- Concurrent use of certain drugs (rifampin, mifepristone, phenytoin, phenobarbital, topiramate, medroxyprogesterone, inhibitors of cortisol synthesis) (double or triple the dose)
- Third trimester of pregnancy (increase by 50%)
- Intercurrent febrile illness (double or triple the dose)
- Minor trauma (double or triple the dose)
- Minor surgery (double or triple the dose)

Parenteral Hydrocortisone Mandatory In:
- Vomiting/diarrhea
- Surgery
- Labor
- Major surgery
- Critical illness (similar to acute crisis management)

Acute Crisis Management
- Measure serum glucose and electrolytes
- Take a blood sample for cortisol, ACTH
- Initiate treatment without waiting for test results
- Intravenous saline (alternate with 5% dextrose if hypoglycemic) 2 to 4 L/24 h
- Intravenous hydrocortisone 100 mg bolus, then
- Intravenous hydrocortisone 100 mg 6-hourly under continuous cardiac monitoring
- Treat underlying cause
- Reduce slowly to 50 mg 6-hourly (after 24 h) then progressive tapering
- Switch to oral replacement (initially double doses, then reduce to standard maintenance dose)

[a] If unavailable use cortisone acetate, 25 to 37.5 mg/d.

Concluding Remarks

Despite significant progress in the understanding and management of CAI, there is still a strong need for the development of better replacement and treatment-monitoring strategies for ACTH deficiency.

REFERENCES

1. Andrioli M, Pecori GF, Cavagnini F. Isolated corticotrophin deficiency. Pituitary 2006;9(4):289–95.
2. Arlt W, Allolio B. Adrenal insufficiency. Lancet 2003;361(9372):1881–93.
3. van Nieuwpoort IC, van Bunderen CC, Arwert LI, et al. Dutch National Registry of GH Treatment in Adults: patient characteristics and diagnostic test procedures. Eur J Endocrinol 2011;164(4):491–7.
4. Webb SM, Strasburger CJ, Mo D, et al. Changing patterns of the adult growth hormone deficiency diagnosis documented in a decade-long global surveillance database. J Clin Endocrinol Metab 2009;94(2):392–9.
5. Stochholm K, Gravholt CH, Laursen T, et al. Incidence of GH deficiency—a nationwide study. Eur J Endocrinol 2006;155(1):61–71.
6. Regal M, Paramo C, Sierra SM, et al. Prevalence and incidence of hypopituitarism in an adult Caucasian population in northwestern Spain. Clin Endocrinol (Oxf) 2001;55(6):735–40.
7. de BH, Blok GJ, Voerman HJ, et al. Body composition in adult growth hormone-deficient men, assessed by anthropometry and bioimpedance analysis. J Clin Endocrinol Metab 1992;75(3):833–7.
8. Johannsson G, Grimby G, Sunnerhagen KS, et al. Two years of growth hormone (GH) treatment increase isometric and isokinetic muscle strength in GH-deficient adults. J Clin Endocrinol Metab 1997;82(9):2877–84.
9. Koltowska-Haggstrom M, Mattsson AF, Shalet SM. Assessment of quality of life in adult patients with GH deficiency: KIMS contribution to clinical practice and pharmacoeconomic evaluations. Eur J Endocrinol 2009;161(Suppl 1):S51–64.
10. Brickman WJ, Silverman BL. Cardiovascular effects of growth hormone. Endocrine 2000;12(2):153–61.
11. Holmes SJ, Economou G, Whitehouse RW, et al. Reduced bone mineral density in patients with adult onset growth hormone deficiency. J Clin Endocrinol Metab 1994;78(3):669–74.
12. Tomlinson JW, Holden N, Hills RK, et al. Association between premature mortality and hypopituitarism. West Midlands Prospective Hypopituitary Study Group. Lancet 2001;357(9254):425–31.
13. Gotherstrom G, Bengtsson BA, Bosaeus I, et al. A 10-year, prospective study of the metabolic effects of growth hormone replacement in adults. J Clin Endocrinol Metab 2007;92(4):1442–5.
14. Wuster C. Fracture rates in patients with growth hormone deficiency. Horm Res 2000;54(Suppl):131–5.
15. Appelman-Dijkstra NM, Claessen KM, Roelfsema F, et al. Long-term effects of recombinant human GH replacement in adults with GH deficiency: a systematic review. Eur J Endocrinol 2013;169(1):R1–14.
16. Mazziotti G, Bianchi A, Bonadonna S, et al. Increased prevalence of radiological spinal deformities in adult patients with GH deficiency: influence of GH replacement therapy. J Bone Miner Res 2006;21(4):520–8.
17. Monson JP. Long-term experience with GH replacement therapy: efficacy and safety. Eur J Endocrinol 2003;148(Suppl 2):S9–14.
18. Svensson J, Bengtsson BA, Rosen T, et al. Malignant disease and cardiovascular morbidity in hypopituitary adults with or without growth hormone replacement therapy. J Clin Endocrinol Metab 2004;89(7):3306–12.
19. Johansson JO, Fowelin J, Landin K, et al. Growth hormone-deficient adults are insulin-resistant. Metabolism 1995;44(9):1126–9.

20. Maison P, Griffin S, Nicoue-Beglah M, et al. Impact of growth hormone (GH) treatment on cardiovascular risk factors in GH-deficient adults: a metaanalysis of blinded, randomized, placebo-controlled trials. J Clin Endocrinol Metab 2004;89(5):2192–9.

21. Cuneo RC, Salomon F, Watts GF, et al. Growth hormone treatment improves serum lipids and lipoproteins in adults with growth hormone deficiency. Metabolism 1993;42(12):1519–23.

22. Claessen KM, Appelman-Dijkstra NM, Adoptie DM, et al. Metabolic profile in growth hormone-deficient (GHD) adults after long-term recombinant human growth hormone (rhGH) therapy. J Clin Endocrinol Metab 2013;98(1):352–61.

23. Sesmilo G, Miller KK, Hayden D, et al. Inflammatory cardiovascular risk markers in women with hypopituitarism. J Clin Endocrinol Metab 2001;86(12):5774–81.

24. Sesmilo G, Biller BM, Llevadot J, et al. Effects of growth hormone administration on inflammatory and other cardiovascular risk markers in men with growth hormone deficiency. A randomized, controlled clinical trial. Ann Intern Med 2000; 133(2):111–22.

25. Markussis V, Beshyah SA, Fisher C, et al. Abnormal carotid arterial wall dynamics in symptom-free hypopituitary adults. Eur J Endocrinol 1997;136(2):157–64.

26. Borson-Chazot F, Serusclat A, Kalfallah Y, et al. Decrease in carotid intima-media thickness after one year growth hormone (GH) treatment in adults with GH deficiency. J Clin Endocrinol Metab 1999;84(4):1329–33.

27. Aimaretti G, Corneli G, Baldelli R, et al. Diagnostic reliability of a single IGF-I measurement in 237 adults with total anterior hypopituitarism and severe GH deficiency. Clin Endocrinol (Oxf) 2003;59(1):56–61.

28. Hartman ML, Crowe BJ, Biller BM, et al. Which patients do not require a GH stimulation test for the diagnosis of adult GH deficiency? J Clin Endocrinol Metab 2002;87(2):477–85.

29. Hoffman DM, O'Sullivan AJ, Baxter RC, et al. Diagnosis of growth-hormone deficiency in adults. Lancet 1994;343(8905):1064–8.

30. Cook DM, Yuen KC, Biller BM, et al. American Association of Clinical Endocrinologists medical guidelines for clinical practice for growth hormone use in growth hormone-deficient adults and transition patients - 2009 update. Endocr Pract 2009;15(Suppl):21–9.

31. Ho KK. Consensus guidelines for the diagnosis and treatment of adults with GH deficiency II: a statement of the GH Research Society in association with the European Society for Pediatric Endocrinology, Lawson Wilkins Society, European Society of Endocrinology, Japan Endocrine Society, and Endocrine Society of Australia. Eur J Endocrinol 2007;157(6):695–700.

32. Maccario M, Valetto MR, Savio P, et al. Maximal secretory capacity of somatotrope cells in obesity: comparison with GH deficiency. Int J Obes Relat Metab Disord 1997;21(1):27–32.

33. Gomez JM, Espadero RM, Escobar-Jimenez F, et al. Growth hormone release after glucagon as a reliable test of growth hormone assessment in adults. Clin Endocrinol (Oxf) 2002;56(3):329–34.

34. Corneli G, Di SC, Baldelli R, et al. The cut-off limits of the GH response to GH-releasing hormone-arginine test related to body mass index. Eur J Endocrinol 2005;153(2):257–64.

35. Chihara K, Shimatsu A, Hizuka N, et al. A simple diagnostic test using GH-releasing peptide-2 in adult GH deficiency. Eur J Endocrinol 2007;157(1):19–27.

36. Popovic V, Leal A, Micic D, et al. GH-releasing hormone and GH-releasing peptide-6 for diagnostic testing in GH-deficient adults. Lancet 2000;356(9236): 1137–42.

37. Drake WM, Coyte D, Camacho-Hubner C, et al. Optimizing growth hormone replacement therapy by dose titration in hypopituitary adults. J Clin Endocrinol Metab 1998;83(11):3913–9.
38. Woodmansee WW, Hartman ML, Lamberts SW, et al. Occurrence of impaired fasting glucose in GH-deficient adults receiving GH replacement compared with untreated subjects. Clin Endocrinol (Oxf) 2010;72(1):59–69.
39. Attanasio AF, Jung H, Mo D, et al. Prevalence and incidence of diabetes mellitus in adult patients on growth hormone replacement for growth hormone deficiency: a surveillance database analysis. J Clin Endocrinol Metab 2011;96(7):2255–61.
40. Luger A, Mattsson AF, Koltowska-Haggstrom M, et al. Incidence of diabetes mellitus and evolution of glucose parameters in growth hormone-deficient subjects during growth hormone replacement therapy: a long-term observational study. Diabetes Care 2012;35(1):57–62.
41. van Bunderen CC, van den Dries CJ, Heymans MW, et al. Effect of long-term GH replacement therapy on cardiovascular outcomes in isolated GH deficiency compared with multiple pituitary hormone deficiencies: a sub-analysis from the Dutch National Registry of Growth Hormone Treatment in Adults. Eur J Endocrinol 2014;171(2):151–60.
42. Burman P, Mattsson AF, Johannsson G, et al. Deaths among adult patients with hypopituitarism: hypocortisolism during acute stress, and de novo malignant brain tumors contribute to an increased mortality. J Clin Endocrinol Metab 2013;98(4):1466–75.
43. Arnold JR, Arnold DF, Marland A, et al. GH replacement in patients with non-functioning pituitary adenoma (NFA) treated solely by surgery is not associated with increased risk of tumour recurrence. Clin Endocrinol (Oxf) 2009;70(3):435–8.
44. Chung TT, Drake WM, Evanson J, et al. Tumour surveillance imaging in patients with extrapituitary tumours receiving growth hormone replacement. Clin Endocrinol (Oxf) 2005;63(3):274–9.
45. Karavitaki N, Warner JT, Marland A, et al. GH replacement does not increase the risk of recurrence in patients with craniopharyngioma. Clin Endocrinol (Oxf) 2006; 64(5):556–60.
46. Charmandari E, Nicolaides NC, Chrousos GP. Adrenal insufficiency. Lancet 2014; 383(9935):2152–67.
47. Hagg E, Asplund K, Lithner F. Value of basal plasma cortisol assays in the assessment of pituitary-adrenal insufficiency. Clin Endocrinol (Oxf) 1987;26(2): 221–6.
48. Nieman LK. Dynamic evaluation of adrenal hypofunction. J Endocrinol Invest 2003;26(Suppl 7):74–82.
49. Cooper MS, Stewart PM. Diagnosis and treatment of ACTH deficiency. Rev Endocr Metab Disord 2005;6(1):47–54.
50. Erturk E, Jaffe CA, Barkan AL. Evaluation of the integrity of the hypothalamic-pituitary-adrenal axis by insulin hypoglycemia test. J Clin Endocrinol Metab 1998;83(7):2350–4.
51. Fiad TM, Kirby JM, Cunningham SK, et al. The overnight single-dose metyrapone test is a simple and reliable index of the hypothalamic-pituitary-adrenal axis. Clin Endocrinol (Oxf) 1994;40(5):603–9.
52. Dorin RI, Qualls CR, Crapo LM. Diagnosis of adrenal insufficiency. Ann Intern Med 2003;139(3):194–204.
53. Borst GC, Michenfelder HJ, O'Brian JT. Discordant cortisol response to exogenous ACTH and insulin-induced hypoglycemia in patients with pituitary disease. N Engl J Med 1982;306(24):1462–4.

54. Stewart PM, Corrie J, Seckl JR, et al. A rational approach for assessing the hypothalamo-pituitary-adrenal axis. Lancet 1988;1(8596):1208–10.
55. Thaler LM, Blevins LS Jr. The low dose (1-microg) adrenocorticotropin stimulation test in the evaluation of patients with suspected central adrenal insufficiency. J Clin Endocrinol Metab 1998;83(8):2726–9.
56. Arlt W. Adrenal insufficiency. Clin Med 2008;8(2):211–5.
57. Howlett TA. An assessment of optimal hydrocortisone replacement therapy. Clin Endocrinol (Oxf) 1997;46(3):263–8.
58. Benson S, Neumann P, Unger N, et al. Effects of standard glucocorticoid replacement therapies on subjective well-being: a randomized, double-blind, crossover study in patients with secondary adrenal insufficiency. Eur J Endocrinol 2012; 167(5):679–85.
59. Arlt W, Callies F, van Vlijmen JC, et al. Dehydroepiandrosterone replacement in women with adrenal insufficiency. N Engl J Med 1999;341(14):1013–20.
60. Allolio B, Arlt W, Hahner S. DHEA: why, when, and how much—DHEA replacement in adrenal insufficiency. Ann Endocrinol (Paris) 2007;68(4):268–73.
61. Johannsson G, Nilsson AG, Bergthorsdottir R, et al. Improved cortisol exposure-time profile and outcome in patients with adrenal insufficiency: a prospective randomized trial of a novel hydrocortisone dual-release formulation. J Clin Endocrinol Metab 2012;97(2):473–81.

Hypophysitis

Hidenori Fukuoka, MD, PhD

KEYWORDS

- Hypophysitis • Autoimmune • CTLA-4 • IgG4 • Hypopituitarism • Diabetes insipidus

KEY POINTS

- Hypophysitis can be classified according to anatomic, histopathologic, and causal criteria.
- Epidemiologic distribution differs according to anatomic classification.
- New categories of this disease have recently been established, such as IgG4-related hypophysitis and secondary hypophysitis caused by anticytotoxic T-lymphocyte antigen-4 antibodies.
- Clinical features can be divided into 4 categories: sellar mass effects, hypopituitarism, central diabetes insipidus, and hyperprolactinemia.
- Clinical management of hypophysitis includes pituitary mass reduction and hormone replacement therapy.

INTRODUCTION

Hypophysitis is characterized by lymphocytic infiltration of the pituitary gland. Depending on the anatomic location of the infiltrate, hypophysitis is classified as lymphocytic adenohypophysitis (LAH), lymphocytic infundibuloneurohypophysitis (LINH), or lymphocytic panhypophysitis (LPH).[1–3] Based on the histopathologic features, there are 2 main forms of hypophysitis (lymphocytic or granulomatous hypophysitis) and 3 rare variants (xanthomatous, IgG4-related, and necrotizing hypophysitis) **(Box 1)**.[1,4–7] This rare infiltration of the pituitary grand occurs mostly in its primary form. However, secondary hypophysitis, presenting as pituitary inflammation, can occur as a symptom of causes such as sellar diseases, systemic diseases, or drugs such as anticytotoxic T-lymphocyte antigen-4 (CTLA-4) antibodies, which have recently been approved for cancer immunotherapy.[1,8] Hypophysitis is also associated with other autoimmune diseases such as Hashimoto thyroiditis, autoimmune polyglandular syndrome (APS), Graves disease, systemic lupus erythematosus, Sjögren syndrome, and type 1 diabetes, reflecting its autoimmune pathogenesis.[1]

The author has nothing to disclose.
Division of Diabetes and Endocrinology, Kobe University Hospital, 7-5-2 Kusunoki-cho, Chuo-ku, Kobe 650-0017, Japan
E-mail address: fukuokah@med.kobe-u.ac.jp

Endocrinol Metab Clin N Am 44 (2015) 143–149
http://dx.doi.org/10.1016/j.ecl.2014.10.011
0889-8529/15/$ – see front matter © 2015 Elsevier Inc. All rights reserved.

> **Box 1**
> **Classification of primary hypophysitis**
>
> 1. Anatomic classification
>
>   Lymphocytic adrenohypophysitis (LAH)
>
>   Lymphocytic infundibuloneurohypophysitis (LINH)
>
>   Lymphocytic panhypophysitis (LPH)
>
> 2. Histopathologic classification
>
>   Lymphocytic hypophysitis
>
>   Granulomatous hypophysitis
>
>   Xanthomatous hypophysitis
>
>   IgG4-related hypophysitis
>
>   Necrotizing hypophysitis
>
>   Mixed forms

EPIDEMIOLOGY

The prevalence and incidence of primary hypophysitis have been estimated mainly from data on surgeries conducted on patients with a pituitary mass or on autoptical specimens. The prevalence of hypophysitis is approximately 0.24% to 0.88%,[1,5,9] and the annual incidence is approximately 1 in 9 million, although this value may be an underestimation.[10] Based on histopathologic classification, the most common form of this disease is lymphocytic hypophysitis (LH; 71.8%), followed by granulomatous hypophysitis (18.6%) and xanthomatous hypophysitis (3.3%), whereas IgG4-related and necrotizing hypophysitis are rare.[5] However, the prevalence of IgG4-related hypophysitis may be underestimated and needs to be clarified.[11] Further characterization is also required for this new entity of hypophysitis, which will improve the definition of the disease.

Hypophysitis generally occurs in the fourth decade of life and is rare in children and the elderly.[12] LAH is 4.3 to 6 times more common in women, especially during late pregnancy and the postpartum period; LINH affects both genders equally, and LPH is more frequent in men (1.8:1).[9,12] The mean age of onset for LAH is lower, particularly in women (women: 35 ± 13 years; men: 45 ± 14 years), than that for other forms (42 ± 17 years).[1] Furthermore, the onset of LPH occurs earlier than that of LINH,[2] and it was even shown to occur at less than 15 years of age for 4 of 34 patients (12%) in 1 study.[2]

RISK FACTORS

Well-known risk factors for primary hypophysitis are pregnancy or childbirth. LAH commonly presents between the last month of gestation and the first 2 months of the postpartum period (57%–69%).[1,12] An additional risk factor for LAH is aseptic meningitis.[13] Several risk factors for secondary forms of hypophysitis have also been identified; these are summarized in **Box 2**.

PATHOPHYSIOLOGY

Table 1 summarizes the pathologic features of hypophysitis.[4,6,11,12,14,15] Antipituitary antibody (APA) is approved for clinical use in indirect immunofluorescence. Patient

Box 2
Factors associated with secondary hypophysitis

1. Seller disease

   Rathke cleft cyst

   Germinoma

   Craniopharyngioma

   Pituitary adenoma

2. Systematic disease

   Wegener granulomatosis

   Langerhans cell histiocytosis

   Giant cell granuloma

   Sarcoidosis

   Takayasu disease

   Crohn disease

   Tuberculosis

   Human immunodeficiency virus

3. Drug

   CTLA-4 blocking antibodies

   Interferon-α

sera are allowed to react with several sections of human surgical specimens, rodent pituitaries, rodent pituitary cell lines, or baboon pituitaries, and antihuman IgG is used as a secondary antibody.[12,16] The sensitivity of APA is 26% to 36% for LAH and 10% for LPH.[1] This antibody reacts positively in 15%, 20%, and 26% of patients with isolated adrenocorticotropic hormone (ACTH), growth hormone, and gonadotropin deficiency, respectively, and in a few patients with isolated thyrotropin deficiency.[17] Because APA has been detected in several other diseases such as type 1 diabetes mellitus, Hashimoto thyroiditis, Graves disease, and pituitary adenomas,

Table 1
Pathologic features of hypophysitis

	Lymphocytic Hypophysitis	Granulomatous Hypophysitis	Xanthomatous Hypophysitis	IgG4-Related Hypophysitis	Necrotizing Hypophysitis
Common feature	Autoimmune infiltration of mainly lymphocytes and plasma cells into the parenchyma of the pituitary gland				
Individual features		Multinucleated giant cells Histiocytes Some forming granulomas findings	Foamy histiocytes (lipid-rich macrophages) Plasma cells Small round mature lymphocytes	Infiltration of IgG4-positive plasma cells Storiform fibrosis	Diffuse necrosis surrounded by dense lymphoplasmacytic infiltrate and few eosinophils

its specificity is poor. Thus, APA is not adequately useful as a diagnostic tool for hypophysitis.[12] However, it could be used as a marker in predicting the future occurrence of hypopituitarism.[16] Several candidates for pathogenic pituitary antibodies have been identified such as those for α-enolase, pituitary gland–specific factors, secretogranin II, T-box transcriptional factor T pit, and intermediate lobe–specific protein.[12,18,19]

With respect to the association between pregnancy and LAH, tumor necrosis factor α (TNF-α) has been shown to cause hypophysitis and is blocked by the placenta-derived soluble TNF receptor 1 protein.[20]

Anti-CTLA-4 antibody treatment, including treatment with ipilimumab and tremelimumab, has been shown to cause hypophysitis in 4.5% of cases.[21] Although the mechanisms remain unknown, this adverse event was identified through injection of the drug into mice, which developed lymphocytic infiltration of the pituitary gland and circulating APA.[22] Investigating the molecular mechanism by which CTLA-4 antibody induces hypophysitis has proved valuable in understanding the pathogenesis of hypophysitis itself.

CLINICAL FEATURES

The clinical features of hypophysitis include sellar mass effects, hypopituitarism, central diabetes insipidus (DI), and hyperprolactinemia.[1,2,9,23,24]

Sellar mass effect induces headaches, visual deficits, and diplopia. Headaches do not correlate with mass volume or its reduction, suggesting that this symptom is not caused only by direct local compression.[1] Visual field deficits occur because of optic chiasm compression and diplopia when masses expand into the cavernous sinus, compressing the III, IV, or VI cranial nerves.[1]

Hypopituitarism is the most prevalent symptom of LAH and LPH, although it is not seen in LINH. The sequential order of trophic hormone deficiency specific to hypophysitis is as follows: ACTH > thyroid-stimulating hormone (TSH) > luteinizing hormone (LH)/follicle-stimulating hormone (FSH) > prolactin (PRL) > growth hormone (GH).[1,9,23–25] On the other hand, in patients with pituitary adenoma or irradiation, the order of hormonal deficiency is: GH > LH/FSH > TSH > ACTH > PRL.[26]

Central DI is characterized by polyuria and polydipsia caused by antidiuretic hormone deficiency.[27] Central DI occurs mainly in LINH and LPH[2]; however, it is also seen in 14% to 20% of patients with sudden-onset LAH.[1,9] Direct inflammatory invasion, destruction, or compression associated with neurohypophysitis might induce central DI in these cases.[28]

Hyperprolactinemia mainly occurs because of stalk compression by the mass; however, direct damage to lactotroph cells, reduced hypothalamic dopamine secretion,[24] and antibodies stimulating the circulation of PRL[1] have also been reported as causes. Hyperprolactinemia can lead to galactorrhea, hypogonadism, amenorrhea, and osteoporosis.[29]

ACUTE MANAGEMENT

The aim of acute management is to decompress the pituitary mass and prevent adrenal crisis. Mass reduction can be achieved through pharmacotherapy, surgery, or irradiation.[1,2,9]

Glucocorticoids can effectively reduce pituitary mass volume. Treatment with prednisone (≥10 mg/d) led to pituitary mass reduction in 62.5% of cases, whereas treatment with lower doses (≤7.5 mg/d) was effective in 44.4% of cases.[30] High doses of methylpredonisolone (120 mg/d for 2 weeks, or 1 g/d for 3 days, followed by a tapering dose) have also been shown to reduce pituitary mass volumes and improve pituitary function.[1,31] In addition, immunosuppressive medications, including azathio-prine, methotrexate, and cyclosporine A, have been used successfully in glucocorticoid-resistant cases.[1]

Surgery is recommended for patients who require diagnostic confirmation or decompression of the optic chiasm. Although surgical intervention is controversial, it is a suitable option for patients with progressive visual deficits, visual acuity, or ocular movement in addition to glucocorticoid resistance.[1] Both stereotactic radiosurgery[32] and stereotactic radiotherapy[1] have been reported to relieve symptoms in patients who show recurrence after surgery and are resistant to glucocorticoids.

CHRONIC MANAGEMENT

The purpose of chronic management in patients with hypophysitis is mainly to restore adequate hormone levels, including those of glucocorticoids, levothyroxine, gonado-tropic or gonadal hormones, GH, and desmopressin. Follow-up studies show that pituitary hormone axis recovery is seen in 41.67% of cases (55.5% for cortisol and 41.67% for gonadotropin), and long-term hormone replacement is required in 73% of hypophysitis cases.[1,23] In granulomatous hypophysitis, panhypopituitarism at presentation predicts a requirement for long-term hormone replacement, whereas galactorrhea, hyperprolactinemia, a normal gonadal axis, and euthyroidism are associated with a reduced requirement.[14] For xanthomatous hypophysitis, improvements in pituitary function after surgical treatment have been shown for less than 50% of cases.[15]

DIFFERENTIAL DIAGNOSES

Hypophysitis can be misdiagnosed as nonfunctioning pituitary adenoma; thus, imaging studies such as MRI are useful tools. Hypophysitis is generally characterized by symmetric enlargement of the pituitary stalk or pituitary gland, with a strong homogeneous gadolinium enhancement. In contrast, pituitary adenomas are asymmetric with stalk displacement and present as less enhanced lesions.[1] Antihypothalamus antibodies have been detected in patients with idiopathic hypopituitarism caused by hypothalamitis, based on reactivity with baboon hypothalamus sections.[33] These antihypothalamus antibodies were colocalized with anti–corticotropin-releasing hormone antibodies in patients with ACTH deficiency or with anti–arginine vasopressin antibodies in patients with central DI.[34]

Anti-Pit-1 antibody syndrome has recently been identified in patients with combined pituitary deficiency, including deficiency of GH, PRL, and TSH.[35] Patients with this syndrome are also predisposed to other autoimmune endocrinopathies, including thyroiditis, adrenalitis, and insulitis, reflecting its relation to APS.

These newly identified categories require further investigation in terms of pathogenesis and prevalence in independent large studies.

PROGNOSIS

Long-term follow-up studies have yet to be performed for patients with hypophysitis. Eleven related deaths from 1962 to 1982 and 14 deaths from 1983 to 2004 have been reported, suggesting that the mortality caused by hypophysitis has not changed despite technological advances.[1] Sudden deaths caused by hypophysitis have been reported for several cases,[36–38] and recurrence after surgical intervention has been noted in 15.3% of cases.[39]

REFERENCES

1. Caturegli P, Newschaffer C, Olivi A, et al. Autoimmune hypophysitis. Endocr Rev 2005;26:599–614.
2. Abe T. Lymphocytic infundibulo-neurohypophysitis and infundibulo-panhypophysitis regarded as lymphocytic hypophysitis variant. Brain Tumor Pathol 2008;25:59–66.
3. Imura H, Nakao K, Shimatsu A, et al. Lymphocytic infundibuloneurohypophysitis as a cause of central diabetes insipidus. N Engl J Med 1993;329:683–9.
4. Leporati P, Landek-Salgado MA, Lupi I, et al. IgG4-related hypophysitis: a new addition to the hypophysitis spectrum. J Clin Endocrinol Metab 2011;96:1971–80.
5. Caturegli P, Iwama S. From Japan with love: another tessera in the hypophysitis mosaic. J Clin Endocrinol Metab 2013;98:1865–8.
6. Shimatsu A, Oki Y, Fujisawa I, et al. Pituitary and stalk lesions (infundibulo-hypophysitis) associated with immunoglobulin G4-related systemic disease: an emerging clinical entity. Endocr J 2009;56:1033–41.
7. Umehara H, Okazaki K, Masaki Y, et al. A novel clinical entity, IgG4-related disease (IgG4RD): general concept and details. Mod Rheumatol 2012;22:1–14.
8. Corsello SM, Barnabei A, Marchetti P, et al. Endocrine side effects induced by immune checkpoint inhibitors. J Clin Endocrinol Metab 2013;98:1361–75.
9. Falorni A, Minarelli V, Bartoloni E, et al. Diagnosis and classification of autoimmune hypophysitis. Autoimmun Rev 2014;13:412–6.
10. Buxton N, Robertson I. Lymphocytic and granulocytic hypophysitis: a single centre experience. Br J Neurosurg 2001;15:242–5 [discussion: 245–6].
11. Bando H, Iguchi G, Fukuoka H, et al. The prevalence of IgG4-related hypophysitis in 170 consecutive patients with hypopituitarism and/or central diabetes insipidus and review of the literature. Eur J Endocrinol 2014;170:161–72.
12. Caturegli P, Lupi I, Landek-Salgado M, et al. Pituitary autoimmunity: 30 years later. Autoimmun Rev 2008;7:631–7.
13. Suzuki K, Izawa N, Nakamura T, et al. Lymphocytic hypophysitis accompanied by aseptic meningitis mimics subacute meningoencephalitis. Intern Med 2011;50:2025–30.
14. Hunn BH, Martin WG, Simpson S Jr, et al. Idiopathic granulomatous hypophysitis: a systematic review of 82 cases in the literature. Pituitary 2013;17(4):357–65.
15. Aste L, Bellinzona M, Meleddu V, et al. Xanthomatous hypophysitis mimicking a pituitary adenoma: case report and review of the literature. J Oncol 2010;2010:195323.
16. Bellastella G, Rotondi M, Pane E, et al. Predictive role of the immunostaining pattern of immunofluorescence and the titers of antipituitary antibodies at presentation for the occurrence of autoimmune hypopituitarism in patients with autoimmune polyendocrine syndromes over a five-year follow-up. J Clin Endocrinol Metab 2010;95:3750–7.
17. Hashimoto K, Yamakita N, Ikeda T, et al. Longitudinal study of patients with idiopathic isolated TSH deficiency: possible progression of pituitary dysfunction in lymphocytic adenohypophysitis. Endocr J 2006;53:593–601.
18. Smith CJ, Bensing S, Burns C, et al. Identification of TPIT and other novel autoantigens in lymphocytic hypophysitis: immunoscreening of a pituitary cDNA library and development of immunoprecipitation assays. Eur J Endocrinol 2012;166:391–8.
19. Smith CJ, Bensing S, Maltby VE, et al. Intermediate lobe immunoreactivity in a patient with suspected lymphocytic hypophysitis. Pituitary 2014;17:22–9.

20. Landek-Salgado MA, Rose NR, Caturegli P. Placenta suppresses experimental autoimmune hypophysitis through soluble TNF receptor 1. J Autoimmun 2012; 38:J88–96.
21. Hodi FS, O'Day SJ, McDermott DF, et al. Improved survival with ipilimumab in patients with metastatic melanoma. N Engl J Med 2010;363:711–23.
22. Iwama S, De Remigis A, Callahan MK, et al. Pituitary expression of CTLA-4 mediates hypophysitis secondary to administration of CTLA-4 blocking antibody. Sci Transl Med 2014;6:230ra45.
23. Khare S, Jagtap VS, Budyal SR, et al. Primary (autoimmune) hypophysitis: a single centre experience. Pituitary 2013. [Epub ahead of print].
24. Rivera JA. Lymphocytic hypophysitis: disease spectrum and approach to diagnosis and therapy. Pituitary 2006;9:35–45.
25. Hashimoto K, Takao T, Makino S. Lymphocytic adenohypophysitis and lymphocytic infundibuloneurohypophysitis. Endocr J 1997;44:1–10.
26. Molitch ME, Clemmons DR, Malozowski S, et al. Evaluation and treatment of adult growth hormone deficiency: an Endocrine Society clinical practice guideline. J Clin Endocrinol Metab 2011;96:1587–609.
27. Oiso Y, Robertson GL, Norgaard JP, et al. Clinical review: treatment of neurohypophyseal diabetes insipidus. J Clin Endocrinol Metab 2013;98:3958–67.
28. Mizokami T, Inokuchi K, Okamura K, et al. Hypopituitarism associated with transient diabetes insipidus followed by an episode of painless thyroiditis in a young man. Intern Med 1996;35:135–41.
29. Melmed S, Casanueva FF, Hoffman AR, et al. Diagnosis and treatment of hyperprolactinemia: an Endocrine Society clinical practice guideline. J Clin Endocrinol Metab 2011;96:273–88.
30. Hashimoto K, Asaba K, Tamura K, et al. A case of lymphocytic infundibuloneurohypophysitis associated with systemic lupus erythematosus. Endocr J 2002; 49:605–10.
31. Kanoke A, Ogawa Y, Watanabe M, et al. Autoimmune hypophysitis presenting with intracranial multi-organ involvement: three case reports and review of the literature. BMC Res Notes 2013;6:560.
32. Ray DK, Yen CP, Vance ML, et al. Gamma knife surgery for lymphocytic hypophysitis. J Neurosurg 2010;112:118–21.
33. De Bellis A, Pane E, Bellastella G, et al. Detection of antipituitary and antihypothalamus antibodies to investigate the role of pituitary or hypothalamic autoimmunity in patients with selective idiopathic hypopituitarism. Clin Endocrinol (Oxf) 2011;75:361–6.
34. De Bellis A, Sinisi AA, Pane E, et al. Involvement of hypothalamus autoimmunity in patients with autoimmune hypopituitarism: role of antibodies to hypothalamic cells. J Clin Endocrinol Metab 2012;97:3684–90.
35. Yamamoto M, Iguchi G, Takeno R, et al. Adult combined GH, prolactin, and TSH deficiency associated with circulating PIT-1 antibody in humans. J Clin Invest 2011;121:113–9.
36. Gal R, Schwartz A, Gukovsky-Oren S, et al. Lymphoid hypophysitis associated with sudden maternal death: report of a case review of the literature. Obstet Gynecol Surv 1986;41:619–21.
37. Gonzalez-Cuyar LF, Tavora F, Shaw K, et al. Sudden unexpected death in lymphocytic hypophysitis. Am J Forensic Med Pathol 2009;30:61–3.
38. Blisard KS, Pfalzgraf RR, Balko MG. Sudden death due to lymphoplasmacytic hypophysitis. Am J Forensic Med Pathol 1992;13:207–10.
39. Leung GK, Lopes MB, Thorner MO, et al. Primary hypophysitis: a single-center experience in 16 cases. J Neurosurg 2004;101:262–71.

Hypopituitarism After Traumatic Brain Injury

Eva Fernandez-Rodriguez, MD[a], Ignacio Bernabeu, MD[a], Ana I. Castro[a,b], Felipe F. Casanueva, MD, PhD[a,b],*

KEYWORDS

- Traumatic brain injury • Hypopituitarism • Growth hormone deficiency
- Hormone replacement therapy

KEY POINTS

- The prevalence of hypopituitarism after traumatic brain injury (TBI) is widely variable in the literature; a meta-analysis that included more than 1,000 patients determined a pooled prevalence of anterior hypopituitarism of 27.5%.
- Growth hormone (GH) deficiency is the most prevalent hormone insufficiency after TBI; however, the prevalence of each type of pituitary deficiency is influenced by the assays used for diagnosis, severity of head trauma, and time of evaluation.
- It is not recommended to evaluate pituitary deficiencies in early acute phases because of the high proportion of pituitary function recovery with the exception of corticotropin deficiency, which should be evaluated within the first several days after TBI.
- Vascular damage and the presence of antipituitary antibodies have been proposed as factors involved in the development of hypopituitarism after TBI.
- Recent studies have demonstrated improvement in cognitive function and cognitive quality of life with substitution therapy in GH-deficient patients after TBI.

INTRODUCTION

TBI is one of the primary causes of death in young people in industrialized countries, and patients who survive suffer important clinical consequences, such as long-term cognitive, behavioral, and social defects.[1,2] TBI represents a significant public health problem worldwide, with a described overall annual incidence in Western countries of 200 to 235 cases per 100,000 individuals.[3]

The authors have nothing to declare.
[a] Endocrinology Division, Departamento de Medicina, Complejo Hospitalario Universitario de Santiago de Compostela, SERGAS, Universidad de Santiago de Compostela, Santiago de Compostela, Spain; [b] Research Centre in Physiopathology of Obesity and Nutrition, Instituto Salud Carlos III, Santiago de Compostela, Spain
* Corresponding author. Endocrinology Division, Hospital Clínico Universitario de Santiago de Compostela, Travesía da Choupana s/n, 15706, Santiago de Compostela, A Coruña, Spain.
E-mail address: endocrine@usc.es

Endocrinol Metab Clin N Am 44 (2015) 151–159
http://dx.doi.org/10.1016/j.ecl.2014.10.012
0889-8529/15/$ – see front matter © 2015 Elsevier Inc. All rights reserved.

endo.theclinics.com

In the past decade, several studies have highlighted the existing relationship between TBI and pituitary dysfunction.[4–15] Hypopituitarism is believed to contribute to TBI-associated morbidity[16] and to functional and cognitive final outcome,[17] neurobehavioral outcome, and quality-of-life impairment.[16] Evaluations have also indicated a specific association between GH deficiency and certain cognitive disorders, such as depression and memory affection.[18] It is also expected that hypopituitarism significantly impedes recovery and rehabilitation after TBI.[19]

PATHOPHYSIOLOGY

The pathophysiology of hypopituitarism after TBI is not completely understood, and several factors implicated in its development have been suggested.[20] One of the main theories involved in pituitary impairment involves vascular damage to the pituitary gland,[21] which is a theory supported by the high prevalence of hypopituitarism in patients who have suffered an ischemic stroke.[22] Vascular damage to the pituitary gland can also be caused by several mechanisms. (1) Traumatic damage to the long hypophyseal portal vessels and subsequent venous infarction are believed to be the main underlying vascular mechanisms.[23,24] The long hypophyseal vessels supply the anterior lobe, which are more susceptible to damage and could explain the higher prevalence of anterior hypopituitarism in cases of TBI. Conversely, the short hypophyseal vessels supply the posterior lobe, which is preserved in most cases and is associated with a lower prevalence of hypopituitarism. (2) Postmortem studies have revealed a high prevalence of necrosis or hemorrhage into the pituitary gland, which suggests a direct traumatic injury to the pituitary gland as another possible mechanism.[25] (3) Multiple secondary insults from hypotension, hypoxia, anemia, and brain swelling could also lead to an ischemic pituitary gland.[26] (4) Another mechanism described as responsible for hypopituitarism due to vascular damage is the transection of the pituitary stalk, which potentially causes hypopituitarism because of infarction of the pituitary tissue.[21,23]

In addition to the vascular damage, recent research has indicated a possible interaction between autoimmunity and the development of hypopituitarism after TBI. It has been demonstrated that antipituitary and antihypothalamic antibodies are present in patients with TBI-induced pituitary dysfunction and persist even 5 years after diagnosis.[27,28] Moreover, in patients with higher titers of pituitary antibodies, the development of pituitary deficiencies is more frequent,[22,29] with increasing importance with a longer duration after trauma.[28] In addition, the recovery of pituitary function is related to negative antibodies titers.[28]

The dynamic condition of hormonal function suggests that head trauma may trigger an ongoing process, such as autoimmunity or neuroinflammation.[30] More studies are still needed, but these findings may support a proposal of the detection of pituitary antibodies as predictive markers of persistent hypopituitarism after TBI.

EPIDEMIOLOGY OF HYPOPITUITARISM AFTER TRAUMATIC BRAIN INJURY

The prevalence of any grade of hypopituitarism after TBI described in published studies thus far is highly variable, ranging from 5.4% to 90%.[4–15,31] In 2007, a meta-analysis, including 1015 patients with TBI, reported a pooled prevalence of hypopituitarism of 27.5%. The prevalence of anterior pituitary dysfunction in the studies included in this meta-analysis ranged from 15% to 68%.[32]

There are no differences in the epidemiology of hypopituitarism in children and adults, with the exception of early childhood. In these cases, the prevalence of pituitary abnormalities is lower and comparable to the prevalence expected for the general population.[33]

The degree and subtype of pituitary deficiencies also varied among the studies published. GH deficiency has been reported as the most prevalent type of pituitary deficiency, particularly as an isolated deficiency,[6,9,10,28] with a prevalence ranging from 2% to 66% and of 28% when the evaluation was performed 5 years after TBI.[28] The prevalence of the other pituitary hormone deficiencies is also widely variable, ranging from 0% to 60% for secondary adrenal insufficiency, 0% to 29% for secondary hypothyroidism, 0% to 29% for central hypogonadism, and 0% to 48% for abnormal hyperprolactinemia.[4–7,9–15,34] Diabetes insipidus tends to improve in long-term survivors, with a reported prevalence of 7% in large series.[35]

There are several explanations for this remarkable variability in the prevalence reported among these studies. The severity of brain damage of the patients, timing of pituitary evaluation, and diagnostic methods used are not homogeneous among the published reports.[34,36]

Severity of Traumatic Brain Injury

TBI severity is graded using the Glasgow Coma Scale (GCS) score[37] according to consciousness level and ocular and motor movements. This scale classifies the head trauma in 3 groups: severe if the score is less than or equal to 8, moderate if the score is from 9 to 12, and mild if the score is greater than or equal to 13.

Pituitary deficiencies have been detected more frequently in cases of moderate and severe trauma (GCS <13),[4,7,12,13,29] although other investigators did not find any association between injury severity and prevalence of hypopituitarism.[5,10,11] The pooled prevalence of hypopituitarism in cases of severe, moderate, and mild TBI reported by Schneider and colleagues in 2007[32] was 35.3, 10.9, and 16.8%, respectively. Several situations, such as the presence of anatomic abnormalities on initial CT scan (diffuse axonal injury or skull fractures),[38] diffuse brain swelling, hypoxia, hypotension,[4] duration of coma,[14] increased intracranial pressure, longer intubation and hospitalization,[32] and advanced age, have been associated with a worse prognosis and predict a higher incidence of hypopituitarism.[39–41] Overall, there is no cost/benefit indication for global screening of all cases of mild TBI.[42] In recent years, however, it has also been reported that sports associated with low-intensity repetitive head trauma may be related to pituitary insufficiency,[43] most likely related to a decrease in pituitary volume,[44] and should be taken in consideration. In these cases, GH deficiency followed by corticotropin deficiency are the most common findings.[44,45]

Timing for Evaluation

Another factor that influences the prevalence of hypopituitarism is the time interval between TBI and pituitary hormone assessment. The design and time of pituitary evaluation in the literature were also variable, ranging from 24 hours up to 23 years after the head trauma. Only a few studies have been designed to evaluate the incidence of hypopituitarism after TBI with specific criteria and evaluation at a particular time,[8,10,13,46] and most of the published studies are retrospective or cross-sectional.[4–7,9,11,15]

The detection of pituitary dysfunction in early acute phases (first 24 h) or acute phases (up to 2–3 weeks) after TBI has not been associated with hypopituitarism after 12 months.[13,46] In 1 study, the prevalence of hypopituitarism was 56% at 3 months but dropped to 36% at 12 months after TBI.[12] This improvement in pituitary function throughout the first year after TBI has been observed particularly in patients with mild and moderate TBI. Conversely, in patients with severe head trauma, pituitary deficiencies may persist even 5 years after the traumatic event.[28] Hypopituitarism has been described as a dynamic condition associated with the development and recovery of hormone deficiencies,[10,13,46] with recovery in pituitary function even 12 years after TBI.[47] Possible pituitary revascularization and cellular pituicyte repopulation may explain these findings.[14]

Moreover, physiologic hormonal changes that can mimic pituitary dysfunction are often observed in the early posttraumatic period.[48] The physiologic response to acute and critical illness comprises hormonal changes similar to GH deficiency, central hypogonadism, and hypothyroidism.[49] Moreover, the metabolism of the protein-binding hormones can be altered by acute illness or drugs frequently used in severe diseases, resulting in increased circulating levels and, consequently, false deficiencies.[50] Conversely, cortisol, prolactin, and vasopressin are stress hormones that are increased in acute phases of severe disease.[51,52] Low or low-normal baseline free cortisol can still be proposed as a potential early marker for the development of chronic corticotropin deficiency in head trauma patients.[48] Acute corticotropin deficiency may be life threatening, and, therefore, the focus during the acute phase should be in detecting glucocorticoid deficiency, with the monitoring of early morning cortisol within the 7 days after TBI in hospitalized patients.[53]

The overestimation of hypopituitarism in the acute phase after TBI makes it reasonable to propose the evaluation of pituitary function at least 1 year after the head trauma and not at an earlier time point, particularly for hormones that do not necessarily need to be replaced urgently, such as the gonadal and somatotropic axes.[54]

Methods for Endocrine Assessment

Another factor that potentially influences the variability in the results reported is the heterogeneity in the methods used for pituitary function evaluation.

The GH axis has been assessed using a dynamic test in addition to basal GH and insulinlike growth factor 1 values. The dynamic tests used, however, have differed among the studies and include the insulin tolerance,[4,15,31,48] glucagon stimulation,[5,11,55] GH-releasing hormone (GHRH)–arginine,[6,10,15] and GHRH–GH-releasing peptide (GHRP)-6[9,13] tests. The vagaries of the GH provocation test are well known.[56] Studies that have used the insulin tolerance test have detected lower prevalence of hypopituitarism.[15,31,57] The optimal diagnostic is the one that identifies the patients who will benefit from treatment with GH and excludes those who will not.[19] The GHRH–GHRP6 test, which is a rigorous and reliable test not affected by known factors that modify GH secretion, such as obesity,[58] has demonstrated its utility in the diagnosis of GH deficiency specifically after TBI,[9,13] even in a single assay after a 30-minute test.[59]

The stimulation tests used when there is a need to evaluate the adrenal axis are the corticotropin stimulation test[7,13] and insulin tolerance test.[4,11,15,60] The corticotropin stimulation test is performed with either 250 μg of cosyntropin[7] or 1 μg of tetracosactrin.[13]

For the thyroid, gonadal, and prolactin axes, basal levels are sufficient for a diagnosis to be made.[7,9,10,15,16,46]

The proposed algorithm for the diagnosis of hypopituitarism after TBI is represented in **Fig. 1**. The recommended tests for diagnosis of hypopituitarism after TBI are the same as for other causes of pituitary dysfunction and have been previously described.[61]

HORMONE REPLACEMENT THERAPY

The Pfizer International Metabolic Database (KIMS) reported a significant improvement in quality of life, as assessed by the Assessment of Growth Hormone Deficiency in Adults score, in patients with posttraumatic hypopituitarism and GH treatment.[62] Recent data also suggest that certain cognitive impairments observed in patients

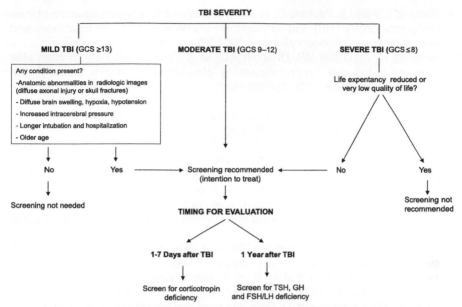

Fig. 1. Proposed algorithm for the diagnosis of hypopituitarism after TBI.

with GH deficiency after TBI and quality of life can improve with GH replacement.[63–65] Serious and life-threatening adrenal crises due to corticotropin deficiency after TBI have significantly improved with glucocorticoid replacement.[60] Long-term follow-up studies are still needed, however, to evaluate the outcome and the necessity and benefits of hormone replacement with GH and gonadal steroids in these patients.

REFERENCES

1. Salazar AM, Warden DL, Schwab K, et al. Cognitive rehabilitation for traumatic brain injury: a randomized trial. Defense and Veterans Head Injury Program (DVHIP) Study Group. JAMA 2000;283(23):3075–81.

2. Khan F, Baguley IJ, Cameron ID. 4: rehabilitation after traumatic brain injury. Med J Aust 2003;178(6):290–5.

3. Tagliaferri F, Compagnone C, Korsic M, et al. A systematic review of brain injury epidemiology in Europe. Acta Neurochir (Wien) 2006;148(3):255–68 [discussion: 268].

4. Kelly DF, Gonzalo IT, Cohan P, et al. Hypopituitarism following traumatic brain injury and aneurysmal subarachnoid hemorrhage: a preliminary report. J Neurosurg 2000;93(5):743–52.

5. Agha A, Rogers B, Sherlock M, et al. Anterior pituitary dysfunction in survivors of traumatic brain injury. J Clin Endocrinol Metab 2004;89(10):4929–36.

6. Bondanelli M, De Marinis L, Ambrosio MR, et al. Occurrence of pituitary dysfunction following traumatic brain injury. J Neurotrauma 2004;21(6):685–96.

7. Lieberman SA, Oberoi AL, Gilkison CR, et al. Prevalence of neuroendocrine dysfunction in patients recovering from traumatic brain injury. J Clin Endocrinol Metab 2001;86(6):2752–6.

8. Aimaretti G, Ambrosio MR, Di Somma C, et al. Traumatic brain injury and subarachnoid haemorrhage are conditions at high risk for hypopituitarism: screening study at 3 months after the brain injury. Clin Endocrinol (Oxf) 2004;61(3):320–6.

9. Popovic V, Pekic S, Pavlovic D, et al. Hypopituitarism as a consequence of traumatic brain injury (TBI) and its possible relation with cognitive disabilities and mental distress. J Endocrinol Invest 2004;27(11):1048–54.

10. Aimaretti G, Ambrosio MR, Di Somma C, et al. Residual pituitary function after brain injury-induced hypopituitarism: a prospective 12-month study. J Clin Endocrinol Metab 2005;90(11):6085–92.

11. Leal-Cerro A, Flores JM, Rincon M, et al. Prevalence of hypopituitarism and growth hormone deficiency in adults long-term after severe traumatic brain injury. Clin Endocrinol (Oxf) 2005;62(5):525–32.

12. Schneider HJ, Schneider M, Saller B, et al. Prevalence of anterior pituitary insufficiency 3 and 12 months after traumatic brain injury. Eur J Endocrinol 2006; 154(2):259–65.

13. Tanriverdi F, Senyurek H, Unluhizarci K, et al. High risk of hypopituitarism after traumatic brain injury: a prospective investigation of anterior pituitary function in the acute phase and 12 months after trauma. J Clin Endocrinol Metab 2006; 91(6):2105–11.

14. Benvenga S, Campenni A, Ruggeri RM, et al. Clinical review 113: hypopituitarism secondary to head trauma. J Clin Endocrinol Metab 2000;85(4):1353–61.

15. Herrmann BL, Rehder J, Kahlke S, et al. Hypopituitarism following severe traumatic brain injury. Exp Clin Endocrinol Diabetes 2006;114(6):316–21.

16. Klose M, Feldt-Rasmussen U. Does the type and severity of brain injury predict hypothalamo-pituitary dysfunction? Does post-traumatic hypopituitarism predict worse outcome? Pituitary 2008;11(3):255–61.

17. Bondanelli M, Ambrosio MR, Cavazzini L, et al. Anterior pituitary function may predict functional and cognitive outcome in patients with traumatic brain injury undergoing rehabilitation. J Neurotrauma 2007;24(11):1687–97.

18. Kelly DF, McArthur DL, Levin H, et al. Neurobehavioral and quality of life changes associated with growth hormone insufficiency after complicated mild, moderate, or severe traumatic brain injury. J Neurotrauma 2006;23(6): 928–42.

19. Blair JC. Prevalence, natural history and consequences of posttraumatic hypopituitarism: a case for endocrine surveillance. Br J Neurosurg 2010;24(1):10–7.

20. Dusick JR, Wang C, Cohan P, et al. Pathophysiology of hypopituitarism in the setting of brain injury. Pituitary 2012;15(1):2–9.

21. Maiya B, Newcombe V, Nortje J, et al. Magnetic resonance imaging changes in the pituitary gland following acute traumatic brain injury. Intensive Care Med 2008;34(3):468–75.

22. Bondanelli M, Ambrosio MR, Carli A, et al. Predictors of pituitary dysfunction in patients surviving ischemic stroke. J Clin Endocrinol Metab 2010;95(10): 4660–8.

23. Daniel PM, Prichard MM, Treip CS. Traumatic infarction of the anterior lobe of the pituitary gland. Lancet 1959;2(7109):927–31.

24. Kornblum RN, Fisher RS. Pituitary lesions in craniocerebral injuries. Arch Pathol 1969;88(3):242–8.

25. Salehi F, Kovacs K, Scheithauer BW, et al. Histologic study of the human pituitary gland in acute traumatic brain injury. Brain Inj 2007;21(6):651–6.

26. Wachter D, Gundling K, Oertel MF, et al. Pituitary insufficiency after traumatic brain injury. J Clin Neurosci 2009;16(2):202–8.

27. Tanriverdi F, De Bellis A, Bizzarro A, et al. Antipituitary antibodies after traumatic brain injury: is head trauma-induced pituitary dysfunction associated with autoimmunity? Eur J Endocrinol 2008;159(1):7–13.

28. Tanriverdi F, De Bellis A, Ulutabanca H, et al. A five year prospective investigation of anterior pituitary function after traumatic brain injury: is hypopituitarism long-term after head trauma associated with autoimmunity? J Neurotrauma 2013; 30(16):1426–33.

29. Schneider HJ, Schneider M, Kreitschmann-Andermahr I, et al. Structured assessment of hypopituitarism after traumatic brain injury and aneurysmal subarachnoid hemorrhage in 1242 patients: the German interdisciplinary database. J Neurotrauma 2011;28(9):1693–8.

30. Tanriverdi F, Unluhizarci K, Kelestrimur F. Persistent neuroinflammation may be involved in the pathogenesis of traumatic brain injury (TBI)-induced hypopituitarism: potential genetic and autoimmune factors. J Neurotrauma 2010;27(2): 301–2.

31. Kokshoorn NE, Smit JW, Nieuwlaat WA, et al. Low prevalence of hypopituitarism after traumatic brain injury: a multicenter study. Eur J Endocrinol 2011;165(2): 225–31.

32. Schneider HJ, Kreitschmann-Andermahr I, Ghigo E, et al. Hypothalamopituitary dysfunction following traumatic brain injury and aneurysmal subarachnoid hemorrhage: a systematic review. JAMA 2007;298(12):1429–38.

33. Heather NL, Jefferies C, Hofman PL, et al. Permanent hypopituitarism is rare after structural traumatic brain injury in early childhood. J Clin Endocrinol Metab 2012; 97(2):599–604.

34. Kokshoorn NE, Wassenaar MJ, Biermasz NR, et al. Hypopituitarism following traumatic brain injury: prevalence is affected by the use of different dynamic tests and different normal values. Eur J Endocrinol 2010;162(1):11–8.

35. Agha A, Thornton E, O'Kelly P, et al. Posterior pituitary dysfunction after traumatic brain injury. J Clin Endocrinol Metab 2004;89(12):5987–92.

36. Gasco V, Prodam F, Pagano L, et al. Hypopituitarism following brain injury: when does it occur and how best to test? Pituitary 2010;15:20–4.

37. Teasdale G, Jennett B. Assessment of coma and impaired consciousness. A practical scale. Lancet 1974;2(7872):81–4.

38. Schneider M, Schneider HJ, Yassouridis A, et al. Predictors of anterior pituitary insufficiency after traumatic brain injury. Clin Endocrinol (Oxf) 2008;68(2): 206–12.

39. Becker DP, Miller JD, Ward JD, et al. The outcome from severe head injury with early diagnosis and intensive management. J Neurosurg 1977;47(4):491–502.

40. Bullock R, Chesnut RM, Clifton G, et al. Guidelines for the management of severe head injury. Brain Trauma Foundation. Eur J Emerg Med 1996;3(2): 109–27.

41. Hellawell DJ, Pentland B. Relatives' reports of long term problems following traumatic brain injury or subarachnoid haemorrhage. Disabil Rehabil 2001;23(7): 300–5.

42. Ghigo E, Masel B, Aimaretti G, et al. Consensus guidelines on screening for hypopituitarism following traumatic brain injury. Brain Inj 2005;19(9):711–24.

43. Tanriverdi F, Unluhizarci K, Karaca Z, et al. Hypopituitarism due to sports related head trauma and the effects of growth hormone replacement in retired amateur boxers. Pituitary 2010;13(2):111–4.

44. Tanriverdi F, Unluhizarci K, Kocyigit I, et al. Brief communication: pituitary volume and function in competing and retired male boxers. Ann Intern Med 2008; 148(11):827–31.

45. Kelestimur F, Tanriverdi F, Atmaca H, et al. Boxing as a sport activity associated with isolated GH deficiency. J Endocrinol Invest 2004;27(11):RC28–32.

46. Tanriverdi F, Ulutabanca H, Unluhizarci K, et al. Three years prospective investigation of anterior pituitary function after traumatic brain injury: a pilot study. Clin Endocrinol (Oxf) 2008;68(4):573–9.

47. Ruggeri RM, Smedile G, Granata F, et al. Spontaneous recovery from isolated post-traumatic central hypogonadism in a woman. Hormones (Athens) 2010; 9(4):332–7.

48. Klose M, Juul A, Struck J, et al. Acute and long-term pituitary insufficiency in traumatic brain injury: a prospective single-centre study. Clin Endocrinol (Oxf) 2007; 67(4):598–606.

49. Van den Berghe G, de Zegher F, Bouillon R. Clinical review 95: acute and prolonged critical illness as different neuroendocrine paradigms. J Clin Endocrinol Metab 1998;83(6):1827–34.

50. Agha A, Ryan J, Sherlock M, et al. Spontaneous recovery from posttraumatic hypopituitarism. Am J Phys Med Rehabil 2005;84(5):381–5.

51. Hamrahian AH, Oseni TS, Arafah BM. Measurements of serum free cortisol in critically ill patients. N Engl J Med 2004;350(16):1629–38.

52. Jochberger S, Morgenthaler NG, Mayr VD, et al. Copeptin and arginine vasopressin concentrations in critically ill patients. J Clin Endocrinol Metab 2006; 91(11):4381–6.

53. Glynn N, Agha A. Which patient requires neuroendocrine assessment following traumatic brain injury, when and how? Clin Endocrinol (Oxf) 2013; 78(1):17–20.

54. Lorenzo M, Peino R, Castro AI, et al. Hypopituitarism and growth hormone deficiency in adult subjects after traumatic brain injury: who and when to test. Pituitary 2005;8(3–4):233–7.

55. Bushnik T, Englander J, Duong T. Medical and social issues related to posttraumatic seizures in persons with traumatic brain injury. J Head Trauma Rehabil 2004;19(4):296–304.

56. Ho KK. Consensus guidelines for the diagnosis and treatment of adults with GH deficiency II: a statement of the GH Research Society in association with the European Society for Pediatric Endocrinology, Lawson Wilkins Society, European Society of Endocrinology, Japan Endocrine Society, and Endocrine Society of Australia. Eur J Endocrinol 2007;157(6):695–700.

57. Klose M, Stochholm K, Janukonyte J, et al. Prevalence of posttraumatic growth hormone deficiency is highly dependent on the diagnostic set-up: results from The Danish National Study on Posttraumatic Hypopituitarism. J Clin Endocrinol Metab 2014;99(1):101–10.

58. Popovic V, Leal A, Micic D, et al. GH-releasing hormone and GH-releasing peptide-6 for diagnostic testing in GH-deficient adults. Lancet 2000;356(9236): 1137–42.

59. Castro AI, Lage M, Peino R, et al. A single growth hormone determination 30 minutes after the administration of the GHRH plus GHRP-6 test is sufficient for the diagnosis of somatotrope dysfunction in patients who have suffered traumatic brain injury. J Endocrinol Invest 2007;30(3):224–9.

60. Agha A, Phillips J, O'Kelly P, et al. The natural history of post-traumatic hypopituitarism: implications for assessment and treatment. Am J Med 2005;118(12): 1416.

61. Sundaram NK, Geer EB, Greenwald BD. The impact of traumatic brain injury on pituitary function. Endocrinol Metab Clin North Am 2013;42(3):565–83.

62. Kreitschmann-Andermahr I, Poll EM, Reineke A, et al. Growth hormone deficient patients after traumatic brain injury–baseline characteristics and benefits after

growth hormone replacement–an analysis of the German KIMS database. Growth Horm IGF Res 2008;18(6):472–8.

63. High WM Jr, Briones-Galang M, Clark JA, et al. Effect of growth hormone replacement therapy on cognition after traumatic brain injury. J Neurotrauma 2010;27(9): 1565–75.
64. Moreau OK, Cortet-Rudelli C, Yollin E, et al. Growth hormone replacement therapy in patients with traumatic brain injury. J Neurotrauma 2013;30(11):998–1006.
65. Reimunde P, Quintana A, Castanon B, et al. Effects of growth hormone (GH) replacement and cognitive rehabilitation in patients with cognitive disorders after traumatic brain injury. Brain Inj 2011;25(1):65–73.

Health-Related Quality of Life in Pituitary Diseases

Iris Crespo, MPsy[a,b], Elena Valassi, MD, PhD[a,b], Alicia Santos, MPsy[a,b],
Susan M. Webb, MD, PhD[a,b],*

KEYWORDS

- Pituitary diseases • Quality of life • Cushing syndrome • Acromegaly • Prolactinoma
- Nonfunctioning pituitary adenoma • Hypopituitarism

KEY POINTS

- Impaired health-related quality of life (QoL) is observed in pituitary diseases.
- Even after endocrine control of acromegaly and Cushing disease, impaired QoL persists.
- Hypopituitarism, affecting 1 or more hormones, tends to worsen QoL further.
- Some physical and psychological factors have been identified as determinants of impaired health-related QoL in patients with pituitary diseases.

INTRODUCTION

Health-related quality of life (QoL) is a concept that refers to individual well-being. It is based on how a particular individual feels, responds, and functions in daily life. Individuals value their QoL, taking into account their expectations, standards, and goals, as well as emotional, physical, and social aspects of their lives, which might be affected if a disease is present.

QoL is usually measured by 2 types of questionnaires: generic and disease-generated or disease-specific. In both, the patients should evaluate how they self-perceive their general health status through several possible ratings (ie, excellent, very good, good, slightly bad, bad). Generic questionnaires have the advantage of being useful in any population, so comparisons can be made between patients with different diseases and normal individuals (**Table 1**). Alternatively, disease-generated

---

The authors have nothing to disclose.

[a] Department of Endocrinology, Hospital Sant Pau, Centro de Investigación Biomédica en Red de Enfermedades Raras (CIBER-ER, Unidad 747), IIB-Sant Pau, ISCIII, Universitat Autònoma de Barcelona (UAB), C/Sant Antoni Maria Claret, n. 167, Barcelona 08025, Spain; [b] Department of Medicine, Hospital Sant Pau, Centro de Investigación Biomédica en Red de Enfermedades Raras (CIBER-ER, Unidad 747), IIB-Sant Pau, ISCIII, Universitat Autònoma de Barcelona (UAB), C/Sant Antoni Maria Claret, n. 167, Barcelona 08025, Spain
* Corresponding author. Department of Endocrinology, Hospital Sant Pau, C/Sant Antoni Maria Claret n.167, Barcelona 08025, Spain.
E-mail address: swebb@santpau.cat

Endocrinol Metab Clin N Am 44 (2015) 161–170
http://dx.doi.org/10.1016/j.ecl.2014.10.013   endo.theclinics.com
0889-8529/15/$ – see front matter © 2015 Elsevier Inc. All rights reserved.

Table 1 Examples of generic and disease-generated questionnaires	
Generic Questionnaires	**Disease-Generated Questionnaires for Pituitary Diseases**
The Nottingham Health Profile[1] The Psychological General Well Being Scale[2] The EuroQol (including the EQ-5 Dimensions and EQ-Visual Analog Scale)[3] The Short Form 36[4]	CushingQoL for Cushing syndrome[5,6] AcroQoL for acromegaly[7] AGHDA (Adult Growth Hormone Deficiency Assessment)[8] or QLS-H (Questions on Life Satisfaction–Hypopituitarism) for growth hormone deficiency[9,10]

questionnaires are more sensitive in identifying dimensions most affected by the disease (eg, improvement after treatment) (see **Table 1**).

Evaluation of a patient's QoL is important to highlight the patient's viewpoint on clinical aspects often not considered by clinicians, to favor a better perception of high-quality medical care, to improve physician-patient relationships, and to contribute to therapeutic decisions based on evidence and cost-efficacy. Moreover, it allows selection of treatments that not only attain biochemical control but also optimize QoL.

CUSHING SYNDROME

The clinical features associated with hypercortisolism in patients with Cushing syndrome (CS) seem to be a strong determinant of well-being and QoL. QoL questionnaires used together with specific evaluations of cognitive functioning or depression have shown impaired QoL in CS, mainly in active patients.[8,11,12] However, cured patients with CS failed to normalize their QoL, even long-term after control of hypercortisolism.[12,13] Complex pharmacologic treatments, need for frequent medical checkups, and concerns about future health deterioration as a result of comorbidity also negatively affect QoL.[13]

Patients with CS most often complain of fatigue/weakness (85%), changes in physical appearance (63%), emotional instability (61%), cognitive problems (mainly poor memory [49%]), depression (32%), and sleeping difficulties (12%).[14] These problems in patients with CS cause negative effects on family life, partner relations, and work/school performance.[14] Furthermore, a retrospective report showed low scores on questions regarding employment status and work capacity in patients with CS both before and after treatment.[15] Although after treatment, 81% of patients with CS were working, 11% were retired because of disability, 5% were retired because of age, and 3% were on sick leave at the time of answering the questionnaire.[15]

The mechanism through which CS determines impairment of QoL is probably multifactorial, involving physical, medical, and psychological factors (**Fig. 1**). Impaired QoL has not been found to correlate with modality of treatment (pituitary or adrenal surgery or pituitary irradiation), duration of follow-up after biochemical remission, disease duration, or severity of hypercortisolism.[8,13] A European-wide study reported that depression was the only negative predictor of the QoL score (using CushingQoL [Cushing Quality of Life Questionnaire]), whereas other variables such as delay to diagnosis, diabetes, or hypertension did not significantly influence it.[16] Patients with CS show more emotional problems (depression and anxiety) and slower recovery after surgery than other patients with pituitary adenomas.[17] Most patients with CS have depression or emotional lability, especially if they are older, women, and have severe hypercortisolism. Psychopathology (mainly atypical depression) was more prevalent

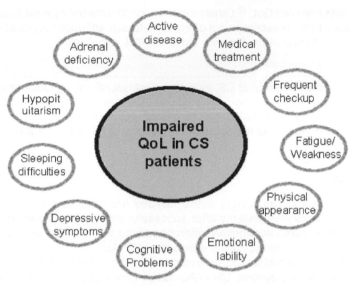

Fig. 1. Factors affecting QoL in patients with CS.

before cure (66.7%) than at 3 months (53.6%), 6 months (36%), and 12 months (24.1%) after successful treatment.[17]

Treatment

Studies mostly agree that there are no differences in QoL between patients with CS of pituitary or adrenal origin, suggesting that persistent QoL deficits after biochemical cure of Cushing disease (CD) are driven by the disease process and hypercortisolism itself, and not by the origin or mode of curative therapy.[6,7,12,16] QoL evaluation after unilateral or bilateral adrenalectomy for CS has shown symptomatic improvement in all patients regardless of their primary diagnosis (adrenal adenoma, CD, ectopic adrenocorticotropic hormone secretion, macronodular hyperplasia, adrenocortical cancer, and pigmented micronodular hyperplasia) and independently of the surgical procedure performed (laparoscopic or open bilateral adrenalectomy), similar to that found in patients treated with pituitary surgery or radiotherapy.[18] When patients with CD were asked to value the impact of adrenalectomy on QoL, 78% (28/36) answered that they had improved, 68% (19/28) referring to a dramatic improvement, but 14% (5/36) experienced no change, and 8% (3/36) stated that their QoL had worsened.[19] Few data comparing pretreatment and posttreatment QoL in patients with CD are available. Vitality/fatigue and general health in the treated group scored better than in the active, pretreatment group, but to a lower degree than seen for the other scales.[20] Fatigue was still present in 46% of treated patients with CD. However, most of these patients (86%) believed that their health status was good to excellent, compared with 1 year before surgery, and 68% reported no problems with moderate activities.[20]

On the other hand, some studies using generic questionnaires, such as the short form 36 (SF-36), showed that pituitary radiotherapy led to greater QoL impairment in patients with CS compared with those who had not been irradiated,[13] but this observation was not confirmed by the CushingQoL questionnaire.[6,7] Wagenmakers and colleagues[12] showed that hormone deficiencies in patients in long-term remission of CS were associated with impaired QoL.[12] Others have not found differences in the CushingQoL score in relation to the presence or not of hypopituitarism, although they described that longer duration of adrenal insufficiency did affect QoL negatively.[6,7]

Summary

Despite successful treatment of CS, long-term residual effects on QoL persist. Complete reversal of physical and psychological comorbidities does not occur immediately after surgery, and poor well-being may be associated with persistence of depressive symptoms, independently of the cause of CS (adrenal or pituitary) and the modality of treatment.

ACROMEGALY

In acromegaly, worse QoL during active disease has persistently been observed compared with controlled patients after successful therapy.[8] However, impairment of QoL persists in cured acromegaly when compared with the normal population or patients with nonfunctioning pituitary adenomas (NFPA).[21]

The impact of the disease and its treatment on the patient's QoL can be great, because of the delay to diagnosis. Lower AcroQoL (Acromegaly Quality of Life Questionnaire) scores in active disease have persistently been observed in different countries, compared with patients in remission, appearance being the most affected and personal relationships the least affected areas. On the other hand, cured patients with acromegaly showed more impairment for physical ability and functioning and more bodily pain than other pituitary tumors like NFPA or prolactinomas.[11] When compared with the general population, SF-36 scores are lower in acromegaly, reflecting impairment of perceived QoL in physical function dimensions but not in the mental ones.[11]

Of the factors affecting QoL, psychological status seems to be one of the most relevant. Acromegaly is associated with higher anxiety-related traits and reduced novelty-seeking behavior and impulsivity, compared with NFPA, which may affect QoL, treatment adherence, and patient-doctor contact.[22] Patients describe themselves as more harm-avoidant and neurotic, and show a high social conformity. Moreover, other factors such as disease duration, active disease, older age, female gender, and presence of joint pain are also negatively correlated with the AcroQoL scores (**Fig. 2**).[23]

Treatment

Pharmacologic decreases lowers growth hormone (GH) and insulin-like growth factor 1 levels and improves both acromegaly comorbidities and QoL.[24] However, the chronic need for monthly injections of somatostatin analogues to control the disease has also been shown to impair AcroQoL scores.[25]

On the other hand, patients treated with radiotherapy have low QoL scores, although it is unknown whether this relates to the more aggressive nature of the disease, which remains active after surgery and medical therapy.[26] Multidisciplinary teams with specific experience in pituitary diseases, including experienced dedicated neurosurgeons, have higher success rates in long-term outcome, and this may improve QoL.[27]

Development of GH deficiency after treatment of acromegaly also affects QoL. The patients least affected were those who attained a normal GH level after treatment (ie, between 0.3 and 1 μg/L), whereas if GH was higher (reflecting active disease), or lower (indicating that these patients had become GH deficient),[28] more impairment ensued. Young adult patients who became GH deficient because of

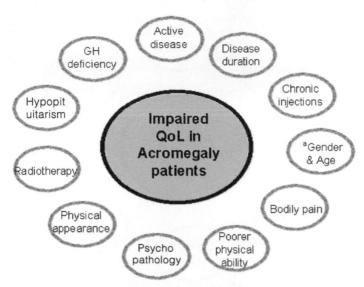

Fig. 2. Factors affecting QoL in patients with acromegaly. [a] Female gender and older age.

previous treatment of acromegaly (with surgery or radiotherapy) improved their QoL, as assessed by the AGHDA (Adult Growth Hormone Deficiency Assessment) questionnaire, after substitution therapy with recombinant human growth hormone (rhGH), but this was not confirmed in older patients.[29]

Summary

QoL is impaired in acromegaly, especially in active disease. This detriment worsens if medical treatment is not provided (with greatest impact on the appearance dimension) and if musculoskeletal symptoms, mainly pain, are present. Other factors, such as psychopathology or GH deficiency, may also affect QoL in these patients.

PROLACTINOMAS

Patients with prolactinomas present poor QoL as evaluated by different generic questionnaires.[11,30–32] Gonadal dysfunction is one of the most important problems in these patients. In men, decreased libido, erectile dysfunction, and poor seminal fluid quality are frequent consequences of prolactin hypersecretion.[33] In women, hyperprolactinemia causes amenorrhea, galactorrhea, vaginal dryness, dyspareunia, and decreased libido, which can lead to infertility.[33] These reproductive dysfunctions have a great impact on the patient's QoL, especially in women (**Fig. 3**).[31]

Mental health and psychological function measures have been described to be impaired in patients with prolactinoma. Altered personality profiles have been reported in these patients compared with the normal population. In particular, patients with prolactinoma presented minor extraversion, lesser novelty seeking, and increased shyness and neuroticism when compared with healthy controls.[32] Moreover, women treated for microprolactinomas have been described as more vulnerable to anxiety and depression symptoms than control individuals.[31]

Treatment

The first-line treatment of prolactinomas, dopamine agonists, are able to reduce tumor size, normalize prolactin levels, and relieve symptoms in these patients,[33] but impaired

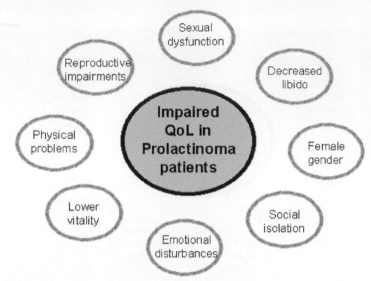

Fig. 3. Factors affecting QoL in patients with prolactinoma.

QoL may persist after successful treatment.[33] Female patients with treated microprolactinoma showed lower scores in physical problems, vitality, emotional aspects, and social isolation compared with control individuals.[30,31] These results were independent of prolactin levels, current or previous intake of dopamine agonists, and dosage or formulation of this treatment.[31]

Summary

Patients with prolactinoma, especially women, show emotional and psychological problems, which negatively affect QoL. It is important to normalize sexual and reproductive function to achieve significant improvement of QoL in these patients. Further insight into these patients' QoL impairment would be possible if a disease-specific questionnaire were available.

NONFUNCTIONING PITUITARY ADENOMAS

Few and conflicting data on QoL in NFPA have been published. Some studies reported that QoL was reduced in treated patients with NFPA,[11,34,35] in contrast with others showing that successful treatment led to normalization of QoL compared with the healthy population.[36] As with prolactinomas, no disease-specific questionnaire is available for these patients with NFPA, which could identify more sensitive or specific impairments in this disease.

In a pilot study, Yedinak and colleagues[37] showed that patients with NFPA expressed greater cognitive dysfunction for mental agility, memory/recall, and verbal recall than patients with acromegaly. However, as well as in the normal population, gender and age seem to be determinants of QoL in patients with NFPA.[34] Patients with NFPA are older than patients with other pituitary adenomas,[11] and recent data indicated that female patients with NFPA have more physical and emotional problems, reduced energy, and poorer health perception compared with their male counterparts (**Fig. 4**).[36]

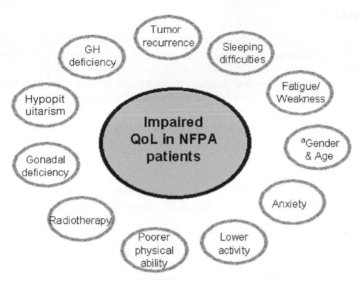

Fig. 4. Factors affecting QoL in patients with NFPA. [a] Female gender and older age.

NFPA adenomas are usually macroadenomas, causing visual field defects, which were associated with reduced interest in leisure activities, without affecting the global QoL score.[35,36] Nonetheless, abnormal scores in physical ability, energy, and anxiety were reported in patients with NFPA with tumor recurrence.[36] Because 20% of tumors relapse 10 years after first surgery, long-term postoperative monitoring is recommended.[38]

Treatment

Disturbed sleep, fatigue, and low motivation have been described in these patients after surgical removal of NFPA.[39] Postoperative hypopituitarism is a strong predictor of reduced QoL.[34,35] In particular, patients with NFPA with hypogonadism reported worse social life and reduced daily activity compared with those having normal gonadotropin function or on correct hormone replacement.[35,36] On the other hand, several studies have found that QoL is impaired in patients suffering GH deficiency,[40] and impairment is worse if other pituitary deficits are present.[41] Patients with NFPA with GH deficiency showed impaired body pain, mental health, and general health perception compared with GH-sufficient patients, which improved after correct replacement with GH.[36] Once treated, improvements can be found in QoL, cardiac function, body composition, and lipid profile.[10,42] Furthermore, patients also have improvements in sexual arousal and body shape after treatment, and have a prompt improvement in dimensions of socializing and tenseness.[43] Some studies also reported that having received radiotherapy can impair mental health or energy levels of patients with NFPA, without affecting their general health perception.[36]

Summary

Specific characteristics of patients with NFPA, such as female gender, hypopituitarism (mainly hypogonadism and GH deficiency), or tumor recurrence seem to be related with impaired QoL. Radiologic and clinical monitoring, hormone replacement, and better sleep quality ameliorate the perception of health status.

HYPOPITUITARISM

Hypopituitarism of either 1 or several pituitary hormones and GH deficiency has been most extensively studied,[40] and impairment is worse if other pituitary deficiencies are also present.[41]

GH deficiency is usually the first pituitary deficiency to appear when hypopituitarism is present, because somatotroph cells are very sensitive to injury. QoL impairment in patients not treated with rhGH increases over time.[44] Conversely, QoL, cardiac function, body composition, and lipid profile improve after substitution therapy with rhGH treatment.[10,42]

Summary

GH deficiency impairs QoL, which improves with substitution therapy with rhGH. Further impairment of QoL can be caused by other concomitant pituitary hormone deficiencies.

REFERENCES

1. Hunt SM, McKenna SP, McEwen J, et al. The Nottingham Health profile: subjective health status and medical consultations. Soc Sci Med 1981;15A:221–9.
2. Ware JE, Snow KK, Kosinski M, et al. SF-36 health survey. manual and interpretation guide. Boston: The Health Institute, New England Medical Center; 1993.
3. Dolan P. Modelling valuations for EuroQol health states. Med Care 1997;35: 1095–108.
4. Gray LC, Goldsmith HF, Livieratos BB, et al. Individual and contextual social-status contributions to psychological well-being. Sociol Soc Res 1983;68:78–95.
5. Webb SM, Badia X, Barahona MJ, et al. Evaluation of health-related quality of life in patients with Cushing's syndrome with a new questionnaire. Eur J Endocrinol 2008;158:623–30.
6. Santos A, Resmini E, Martínez-Momblán MA, et al. Psychometric performance of the CushingQoL questionnaire in conditions of clinical practice. Eur J Endocrinol 2012;167:337–42.
7. Webb SM, Prieto L, Badia X, et al. Acromegaly Quality of Life Questionnaire (ACROQOL) a new health-related quality of life questionnaire for patients with acromegaly: development and psychometric properties. Clin Endocrinol 2002; 57:251–8.
8. McKenna SP, Doward LC, Alonso J, et al. The QoL.AGHDA: an instrument for the assessment of quality of life in adults with growth hormone deficiency. Qual Life Res 1999;8:373–83.
9. Blum WF, Shavrikova EP, Edwards DJ, et al. Decreased quality of life in adult patients with growth hormone deficiency compared with general populations using the new, validated, self-weighted questionnaire, questions on life satisfaction hypopituitarism module. J Clin Endocrinol Metab 2003;88:4158–67.
10. Rosilio M, Blum WF, Edwards DJ, et al. Long-term improvement of quality of life during growth hormone (GH) replacement therapy in adults with GH deficiency, as measured by questions on life satisfaction-hypopituitarism (QLS-H). J Clin Endocrinol Metab 2004;89:1684–93.
11. Johnson MD, Woodburn CJ, Vance ML. Quality of life in patients with a pituitary adenoma. Pituitary 2003;6:81–7.
12. Wagenmakers MA, Netea-Maier RT, Prins JB, et al. Impaired quality of life in patients in long-term remission of Cushing's syndrome of both adrenal and pituitary

origin: a remaining effect of long-standing hypercortisolism? Eur J Endocrinol 2012;167:687–95.

13. Van Aken MO, Pereira AM, Biermasz NR, et al. Quality of life in patients after long-term biochemical cure of Cushing's disease. J Clin Endocrinol Metab 2002;90: 3279–86.

14. Gotch PM. Cushing's syndrome from the patient's perspective. Endocrinol Metab Clin North Am 1994;23:607–17.

15. Pikkarainen L, Sane T, Reunanen A. The survival and well-being of patients treated for Cushing's syndrome. J Intern Med 1999;245:463–8.

16. Valassi E, Santos A, Yaneva M, et al. The European Registry on Cushing's syndrome: 2-year experience. Baseline demographic and clinical characteristics. Eur J Endocrinol 2011;165:383–92.

17. Dorn LD, Burgess ES, Friedman TC, et al. The longitudinal course of psychopathology in Cushing's syndrome after correction of hypercortisolism. J Clin Endocrinol Metab 1997;82:912–9.

18. Thompson SK, Hayman AV, Ludlam WH, et al. Improved quality of life after bilateral laparoscopic adrenalectomy for Cushing's disease: a 10-year experience. Ann Surg 2007;245:790–4.

19. Sippel RS, Elaraj DM, Kebebew E, et al. Waiting for change: symptom resolution after adrenalectomy for Cushing's syndrome. Surgery 2008;144:1054–61.

20. Smith PW, Turza KC, Carter CO, et al. Bilateral adrenalectomy for refractory Cushing's Disease: a safe and definitive therapy. J Am Coll Surg 2009;208: 1059–64.

21. Tiemensma J, Kaptein AA, Pereira AM, et al. Affected illness perceptions and the association with impaired quality of life in patients with long-term remission of acromegaly. J Clin Endocrinol Metab 2011;96(11):3550–8.

22. Sievers C, Ising M, Pfister H, et al. Personality in patients with pituitary adenomas is characterized by increased anxiety related traits: comparison of 70 acromegalic patients to patients with non-functioning pituitary adenomas and age and gender matched controls. Eur J Endocrinol 2009;160:367–73.

23. Miller A, Doll H, David J, et al. Impact of musculoskeletal disease on quality of life in long-standing acromegaly. Eur J Endocrinol 2008;158:587–93.

24. Neggers SJ, van Aken MO, de Herder WW, et al. Quality of life in acromegalic patients during long-term somatostatin analog treatment with and without pegvisomant. J Clin Endocrinol Metab 2008;93:3853–9.

25. Postma MR, Netea-Maiter RT, Van den Berg G, et al. Quality of life is impaired in association with the need for prolonged postoperative therapy by somatostatin analogs in patients with acromegaly. Eur J Endocrinol 2012;166:585–92.

26. Van der Klaauw AA, Biermasz NR, Hoftijzer HC, et al. Previous radiotherapy negatively influences quality of life during 4 years of follow-up in patients cured from acromegaly. Clin Endocrinol (Oxf) 2008;69:123–8.

27. Bates PR, Carson MN, Trainer PJ, et al. Wide variation in surgical outcomes for acromegaly in the UK. Clin Endocrinol (Oxf) 2008;68:136–42.

28. Kauppinen-Mäkelin R, Sane T, Sintonen H, et al. Quality of life in treated patients with acromegaly. J Clin Endocrinol Metab 2006;91:3891–6.

29. Wexler T, Gunnell L, Omer Z, et al. Growth hormone deficiency is associated with decreased quality of life in patients with prior acromegaly. J Clin Endocrinol Metab 2009;94:2471–7.

30. Cesar de Oliveira Naliato E, Dutra Violante AH, Caldas D, et al. Quality of life in women with microprolactinoma treated with dopamine agonists. Pituitary 2008; 11:247–54.

31. Kars M, van der Klaauw AA, Onstein CS, et al. Quality of life is decreased in female patients treated for microprolactinoma. Eur J Endocrinol 2007;157:133–9.
32. Athanasoulia AP, Ising M, Pfister H, et al. Distinct dopaminergic personality patterns in patients with prolactinomas: a comparison with non-functioning pituitary adenoma patients and age- and gender-matched controls. Neuroendocrinology 2012;96:204–11.
33. Kars M, Dekkers OM, Pereira AM, et al. Update in prolactinomas. Neth J Med 2010;68:104–12.
34. Van der Klaauw AA, Kars M, Biermasz NR, et al. Disease-specific impairments in quality of life during long-term follow-up of patients with different pituitary adenomas. Clin Endocrinol 2008;69:775–84.
35. Dekkers OM, van der Klaauw AA, Pereira AM, et al. Quality of life is decreased after treatment for nonfunctioning pituitary macroadenomas. J Clin Endocrinol Metab 2006;91:3364–9.
36. Capatina C, Christodoulides C, Fernandez A, et al. Current treatment protocols can offer a normal or near normal quality of life in the majority of patients with non-functioning pituitary adenomas. Clin Endocrinol 2013;78:86–93.
37. Yedinak CG, Fleseriu M. Self-perception of cognitive function among patients with active acromegaly, controlled acromegaly, and non-functional pituitary adenoma: a pilot study. Endocrine 2014;46(3):585–93.
38. Reddy R, Cudlip S, Byrne JV, et al. Can we ever stop imaging in surgically treated and radiotherapy-naive patients with non-functioning pituitary adenoma? Eur J Endocrinol 2011;165:739–44.
39. Biermasz NR, Joustra SD, Donga E, et al. Patients previously treated for non-functioning pituitary macroadenomas have disturbed sleep characteristics, circadian movement rhythm and subjective sleep quality. J Clin Endocrinol Metab 2011;96:1524–32.
40. Cuneo R, Salomon F, McGauley G, et al. The growth hormone deficiency syndrome in adults. Clin Endocrinol 1992;37:387–97.
41. Koltowska-Häggström M, Kind P, Monson, et al. Growth hormone (GH) replacement in hypopituitary adults with GH deficiency evaluated by a utility-weighted quality of life index: a precursor to cost-utility analysis. Clin Endocrinol 2008;68:122–9.
42. Giavoli C, Profka E, Verrua E, et al. GH replacement improves quality of life and metabolic parameters in cured acromegalic patients with growth hormone deficiency. J Clin Endocrinol Metab 2012;97:3983–8.
43. Koltowska-Häggström M, Mattsson AF, Shalet SM. Assessment of quality of life in adult patients with GH deficiency: KIMS contribution to clinical practice and pharmacoeconomic evaluations. Eur J Endocrinol 2009;161(Suppl 1):S51–64.
44. Gilchrist FJ, Murray RD, Shalet SM. The effect of long-term untreated growth hormone deficiency (GHD) and 9 years of GH replacement on the quality of life (QoL) of GH-deficient adults. Clin Endocrinol 2002;57:363–70.

Pituitary Diseases and Bone

Gherardo Mazziotti, MD, PhD, Silvia Chiavistelli, MD, Andrea Giustina, MD*

KEYWORDS

- Pituitary diseases • Osteoporosis • Bone mineral density • Fractures
- Growth hormone • Prolactin • Cortisol • Sex steroids

KEY POINTS

- Fragility fractures are frequent complications of pituitary diseases.
- Deficiency and excess of growth hormone may be cause of skeletal fragility.
- Overtreatment of central hypoadrenalism and hypothyroidism may contribute to an increased fracture risk in patients with hypopituitarism.
- In pituitary diseases, the occurrence of vertebral fractures is not strictly dependent on bone mineral density.

INTRODUCTION

The skeleton is an extremely dynamic tissue with a continuous remodeling process guided by bone-forming osteoblasts and bone-resorbing osteoclasts.[1] The traditional paradigm is that pituitary-derived hormones exert their biological effects on bone by peripheral mediators produced by target glands under their stimulation. However, pituitary hormones have been also shown to bypass peripheral endocrine organs, possibly exerting remarkable direct effects on the skeleton (**Fig. 1**).[2–10]

SKELETAL FRAGILITY IN PITUITARY DISEASES: CLINICAL AND THERAPEUTIC ASPECTS
Prolactin-Secreting Adenomas

Patients with prolactinomas have high bone turnover (**Box 1**), with uncoupling between bone resorption and bone formation markers in some experiences.[11] This uncoupled bone turnover may explain the bone loss, with osteopenia and osteoporosis occurring predominantly at the lumbar spine[12] in association with hypogonadism, duration of disease, serum values of prolactin (PRL), and bone turnover markers.[13,14] Patients with prolactinomas may develop vertebral and nonvertebral fractures.[15–17] A high prevalence of morphometric vertebral fractures[18] (**Box 2**) was

The authors have nothing to disclose.
Endocrinology, University of Brescia, Via Biseo 17, Brescia 25123, Italy
* Corresponding author.
E-mail address: a.giustina@libero.it

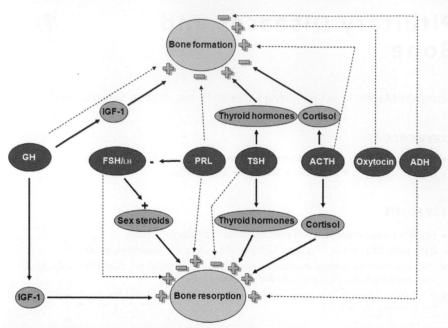

Fig. 1. Direct and indirect effects of pituitary hormones on bone remodeling. ACTH, cortico-tropin; +, positive effect; −, negative effect; ADH, antidiuretic hormone/vasopressin; dashed line, suggested effect; FSH, follicle-stimulating hormone; GH, growth hormone; IGF-1, insu-lin-like growth factor 1; LH, luteinizing hormone; PRL, prolactin; solid line, well-demonstrated effect; TSH, thyrotropin.

Box 1
Bone turnover in pituitary diseases

Suppression of bone turnover

   Growth hormone deficiency

   Cushing disease

   Overtreatment of central hypoadrenalism

Increase of bone turnover

   Acromegaly

   Hypogonadism

   Prolactinomas

   Overtreatment of central hypothyroidism

Box 2
Morphometric classification of radiologic vertebral fractures

Vertebral fractures are identified by marking the vertebral body with 6 points to describe the vertebral shape and heights. According to the quantitative morphometric approach, vertebral fractures are defined as mild, moderate, and severe, based on a height ratio decrease of 20% to 25%, 25% to 40%, and more than 40%, respectively.

> **Box 3**
> **Direct effects of prolactin (PRL) on bone remodeling**
>
> - PRL receptor was demonstrated in osteoblasts
> - PRL was shown to decrease in vitro osteoblast proliferation with a secondary impairment of bone formation and mineralization
> - PRL induced an increase in receptor activator of nuclear factor-kb ligand/osteoprotegerin expression in osteoblasts, leading to an increase in bone resorption

reported even in postmenopausal women with prolactinomas[17] and in men with normal testosterone values,[16] supporting the hypothesis that PRL excess per se may contribute to skeletal fragility (**Box 3**). The frequency of vertebral fractures was significantly associated with duration of disease independently of the effects of hypopituitarism, age of the patients, and serum PRL levels.[17] Patients with fractures were shown to have lower bone mineral density (BMD) than those without fractures as measured by dual x-ray absorptiometry (DXA), but only a minority of patients had either osteoporosis or BMD below the expected range for age.[16,17]

Treatment of prolactinomas with dopaminergic drugs was shown to improve BMD,[19] although some studies reported only partial recovery of osteopenia and osteoporosis in patients with prolactinomas.[11] There are no prospective studies investigating the outcome of fracture risk after treatment of prolactinomas. Few data from cross-sectional studies suggest that correction of hyperprolactinemia may lead to a significant decrease of fracture risk in women with prolactinomas, although there is also evidence that fracture risk may remain high in some patients, especially if male and/or with long-standing hyperprolactinemia, independently of medical treatment.[16]

Growth Hormone–Secreting Adenomas

Consistently with the concept that excess growth hormone (GH) stimulates bone remodeling (**Box 4; Fig. 2**), markers of bone formation and resorption are increased in patients with active acromegaly (see **Box 1**), whereas data on BMD are somewhat variable in relation to the skeletal site, activity of disease, and gonadal status.[2] However, other factors may also underlie this variability (**Box 5**).

Although BMD is not consistently decreased, there is convincing evidence that acromegaly causes impairment of vertebral resistance in affected patients with high risk of vertebral fractures.[20–28] According to the accumulated data in the literature, radiologic vertebral fractures (see **Box 2**) may occur in more than one-third of

> **Box 4**
> **Effects of growth hormone (GH) on bone remodeling**
>
> - GH stimulates the proliferation of cells of the osteoblastic lineage and affects the fate of mesenchymal precursors, favoring osteoblastogenesis and chondrogenesis and opposing adipogenesis
> - GH stimulates, either directly or indirectly through insulin-like growth factor 1 (IGF-1), the differentiated function of mature osteoblasts
> - GH also stimulates the carboxylation of osteocalcin, which is a marker of osteoblastic function, and stimulates production of receptor activator of nuclear factor-kb ligand and osteoprotegerin

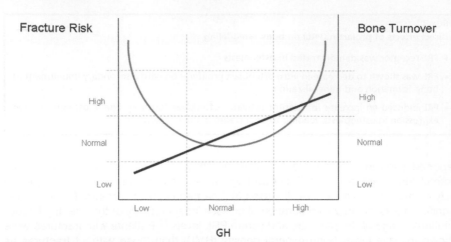

Fig. 2. U-shape curve of the fracture risk in correlation with growth hormone (GH) levels and consequent changes in bone turnover.

acromegaly patients (**Table 1**). The occurrence of vertebral fractures in acromegaly correlated with the duration of active disease and levels of serum insulin-like growth factor 1 (IGF-I) (see **Fig. 2**), but not with BMD, as they were found to develop even in patients with normal or minimally decreased BMD.[20,23] Appropriate and effective treatment of acromegaly improves skeletal health,[27] although the risk of vertebral fractures may persist as high in some patients with well-controlled or cured acromegaly in relation with preexistent vertebral fractures and untreated hypogonadism.[27,28] Therefore, guidelines for the diagnosis and follow-up of acromegaly complications now include not only DXA[29] but also evaluation of the spine by morphometric radiography (see **Box 2**).[18,30]

Corticotropin-Secreting Adenomas

Skeletal fragility is a frequent complication of Cushing disease.[6] When the disease is diagnosed, the skeletal phenotype is usually characterized by a low bone turnover (see **Box 1**) with a slight and uncoupled increase in bone resorption (for detailed mechanistic reviews, please refer to Canalis and colleagues[31]). BMD may be normal or only slightly decreased, whereas fracture risk increases rapidly after few months of exposure to endogenous hypercortisolism.[6] In fact, fragility fractures may be the first clinical manifestation of Cushing disease.[32] Fractures more frequently involve the

---

Box 5
Factors affecting bone mineral density (BMD) values in patients with acromegaly

- Patients with acromegaly are frequently affected by osteoarthritis with structural modifications of the spine consisting in osteophyte formation and facet-joint hypertrophy, which may lead to an overestimation of BMD measured at the lumbar spine

- Excess GH and IGF-1 may exert a deleterious effect on trabecular microarchitecture, whereas cortical bone density tends to be increased as effect of GH on periosteal ossification

- Dual x-ray absorptiometry does not distinguish between cortical and trabecular bone, and densitometric results are greatly influenced by the variable distribution of these 2 compartments in the different skeletal sites

Table 1
Studies investigating the prevalence (P) and incidence (I) of vertebral fractures in acromegaly

Authors,[Ref.] Year	Study Design	Patients n	Mean/Median Age y	Sex M/F	Active Disease %	Hypogonadism %	Vertebral Fractures %
Bonadonna et al,[20] 2005	Cross-sectional	36	61	0/36	42	100	53(P)
Mazziotti et al,[21] 2008	Cross-sectional	40	47	40/0	63	33	57(P)
Battista et al,[22] 2009	Retrospective	46	51	23/23	48	50	28(P)
Wassenaar et al,[23] 2011	Cross-sectional	89	58	46/43	0	52	59(P)
Padova et al,[24] 2011	Cross-sectional	18	47	8/12	60	50	39(P)
Madeira et al,[25] 2013	Cross-sectional	75	56	22/53	72	44	11(P)
Brzana et al,[26] 2014	Retrospective	32	48	23/9	0	50	37(P)
Mazziotti et al,[27] 2013	Prospective	88	50	55/33	46	28	42(I)
Claessen et al,[28] 2013	Prospective	49	61	18/31	0	35	20(I)
Overall		473					38

Data from Refs.[20–28]

vertebrae and may occur in 30% to 50% of patients with Cushing disease, in close association with the severity of hypercortisolism.[6,33]

Bone health does not always completely recover after correction of endogenous hypercortisolism.[34] In fact, some patients may experience an increase in bone formation soon after resolution of glucocorticoid excess with secondary improvement of BMD and a decrease in fracture risk,[35] whereas in other patients the risk of fracture continue to remain high over the long term after the cure of disease,[36] needing personalized treatment with bone-active drugs.[37]

Hypopituitarism

Low bone turnover and decreased BMD is reported in patients with GH deficiency (GHD) (see **Box 1**), either isolated or combined with other pituitary hormone deficiencies.[38] The degree of bone loss is related to the duration and age of onset of GHD, the severity of the disease, and the age of the patients. About half of the patients have normal vertebral BMD.[2] In childhood-onset GHD, vertebral BMD is reduced with T scores often between −1 and −2; about one-third of the patients have T scores of −2.5 or less.[39] By contrast, patients with adult-onset GHD often have normal vertebral T scores. The reasons for the different degrees of bone loss may be the occurrence of childhood-onset GHD before the achievement of peak bone mass and the longer disease duration (underestimation of BMD may be also related to low size and volume of bones in short-stature patients with GHD[40]). The degree of bone loss in adult-onset GHD inversely correlated with age (eg, lower BMD in younger patients) and positively with duration and severity of the disease.[41] Data on fractures in GHD are limited.[42–45] Prevalent morphometric vertebral fractures[18] (see **Box 2**) were found in more than 50% of adult patients with GHD (in about one-third of whom fractures were moderate to severe; see **Box 2**).[44] Vertebral fractures were shown to occur even in hypopituitary patients with normal BMD.[44]

Because GHD is the main determinant of skeletal fragility in patients with hypopituitarism, treatment with recombinant human GH (rhGH) is expected to induce positive effects on the skeleton. Most of the trials performed so far have suggested that rhGH had a biphasic effect on bone, because after an initial (6–12 months) predominance of bone resorption, stimulation of formation became predominant when treatment was continued for longer periods of time.[46] Consistently with this biphasic effect on bone remodeling, a beneficial effect of rhGH therapy on lumbar spine and femoral neck BMD was demonstrated only in studies longer than 12 months.[47] Along with the effects on BMD, rhGH replacement therapy was also shown to improve muscle performance, which may contribute toward decreasing the risk of fracture in this clinical context.[48]

Box 6
Effects of overreplacement of hypopituitarism on vertebral fractures

- Higher prevalence of vertebral fractures was demonstrated in hypopituitary patients treated with hydrocortisone doses greater than 28 mg per day

- The negative effects of glucocorticoid overtreatment were shown to be more evident in patients with untreated GH deficiency

- Higher prevalence of vertebral fractures was demonstrated in hypopituitary patients treated with thyroxine doses greater than 1.35 µg/kg per day

- The negative skeletal effects of thyroxine overtreatment were more evident in patients with replaced GH deficiency

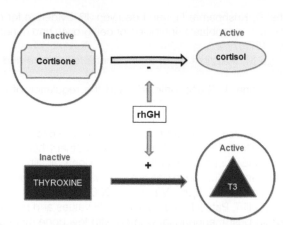

Fig. 3. Interplay between recombinant human growth hormone (rhGH) therapy and peripheral metabolism of cortisone and thyroxine. +, positive effect; −, negative effect; T3, triiodiothyronine.

Therapeutic data on fractures are scanty and limited to cross-sectional observations showing lower prevalence of vertebral fractures in patients who started rhGH treatment early after diagnosis of GHD.[44]

Replacement therapies of central hypoadrenalism and hypothyroidism were shown to influence the fracture rate in patients with hypopituitarism[49,50] in association with untreated or treated GHD, respectively (**Box 6; Fig. 3**). In fact, overtreatment with these hormones may be frequent in patients with hypopituitarism because replacement therapies do not completely mirror the endogenous hormonal production, and their monitoring is also made difficult by the lack of good biomarkers of their action.

SUMMARY

Vertebral fractures are frequent and still largely underestimated complications of pituitary diseases occurring even in patients with normal BMD. Therefore, morphometric radiographic evaluation of the spine should always be considered when monitoring of these patients is planned. Although treatment of pituitary hormone excess or defect generally improves skeletal health, some patients with cured pituitary diseases may still have a high risk of fracture, providing the rationale to use bone-active drugs in this specific clinical setting.

REFERENCES

1. Mazziotti G, Bilezikian J, Canalis E, et al. New understanding and treatments for osteoporosis. Endocrine 2012;41:58–69.
2. Giustina A, Mazziotti G, Canalis E. Growth hormone, insulin-like growth factors, and the skeleton. Endocr Rev 2008;29:535–59.
3. Iqbal J, Blair HC, Zallone A, et al. Further evidence that FSH causes bone loss independently of low estrogen. Endocrine 2012;412:171–5.
4. Omodei U, Mazziotti G, Donarini G, et al. Effects of recombinant follicle-stimulating hormone on bone turnover markers in infertile women undergoing in vitro fertilization procedure. J Clin Endocrinol Metab 2013;981:330–6.

5. Seriwatanachai D, Krishnamra N, van Leeuwen JP. Evidence for direct effects of prolactin on human osteoblasts: inhibition of cell growth and mineralization. J Cell Biochem 2009;107:677–85.

6. Mancini T, Doga M, Mazziotti G, et al. Cushing's syndrome and bone. Pituitary 2004;7:249–52.

7. Mazziotti G, Giustina A. Glucocorticoids and the regulation of growth hormone secretion. Nat Rev Endocrinol 2013;95:265–76.

8. Giustina A, Wehrenberg WB. Influence of thyroid hormones on the regulation of growth hormone secretion. Eur J Endocrinol 1995;133:646–53.

9. Mazziotti G, Sorvillo F, Piscopo M, et al. Recombinant human TSH modulates in vivo C-telopeptides of type-1 collagen and bone alkaline phosphatase, but not osteoprotegerin production in postmenopausal women monitored for differentiated thyroid carcinoma. J Bone Miner Res 2005;20:480–6.

10. Mazziotti G, Porcelli T, Patelli I, et al. Serum TSH values and risk of vertebral fractures in euthyroid post-menopausal women with low bone mineral density. Bone 2010;46:747–51.

11. Di Somma C, Colao A, Di Sarno A, et al. Bone marker and bone density responses to dopamine agonist therapy in hyperprolactinemic males. J Clin Endocrinol Metab 1998;83:807–13.

12. Naliato EC, Violante AH, Caldas D, et al. Bone density in women with prolactinoma treated with dopamine agonists. Pituitary 2008;11(1):21–8.

13. Colao A, Di Somma C, Loche S, et al. Prolactinomas in adolescents: persistent bone loss after 2 years of prolactin normalization. Clin Endocrinol 2000;52:319–27.

14. Klibanski A, Biller BM, Rosenthal DI, et al. Effects of prolactin and estrogen deficiency in amenorrheic bone loss. J Clin Endocrinol Metab 1988;67:124–30.

15. Vestergaard P, Jørgensen JO, Hagen C, et al. Fracture risk is increased in patients with GH deficiency or untreated prolactinomas—a case-control study. Clin Endocrinol (Oxf) 2002;56(2):159–67.

16. Mazziotti G, Porcelli T, Mormando M, et al. Vertebral fractures in males with prolactinoma. Endocrine 2011;39:288–93.

17. Mazziotti G, Mancini T, Mormando M, et al. High prevalence of radiological vertebral fractures in women with prolactin-secreting pituitary adenomas. Pituitary 2011;14(4):299–306.

18. Griffith JF, Genant HK. New advances in imaging osteoporosis and its complications. Endocrine 2012;42:39–51.

19. Klibanski A, Greenspan SL. Increase in bone mass after treatment of hyperprolactinemic amenorrhea. N Engl J Med 1986;315:542–6.

20. Bonadonna S, Mazziotti G, Nuzzo M, et al. Increased prevalence of radiological spinal deformities in active acromegaly: a cross-sectional study in postmenopausal women. J Bone Miner Res 2005;20:1837–44.

21. Mazziotti G, Bianchi A, Bonadonna S, et al. Prevalence of vertebral fractures in men with acromegaly. J Clin Endocrinol Metab 2008;93:4649–55.

22. Battista C, Chiodini I, Muscarella S, et al. Spinal volumetric trabecular bone mass in acromegalic patients: a longitudinal study. Clin Endocrinol 2009;70:378–82.

23. Wassenaar MJ, Biermasz NR, Hamdy NA, et al. High prevalence of vertebral fractures despite normal bone mineral density in patients with long-term controlled acromegaly. Eur J Endocrinol 2011;164:475–83.

24. Padova G, Borzì G, Incorvaia L, et al. Prevalence of osteoporosis and vertebral fractures in acromegalic patients. Clin Cases Miner Bone Metab 2011;8:37–43.

25. Madeira M, Neto LV, Torres CH, et al. Vertebral fracture assessment in acromegaly. J Clin Densitom 2013;16:238–43.

26. Brzana J, Yedinak CG, Hameed N, et al. FRAX score in acromegaly: does it tell the whole story? Clin Endocrinol 2014;80:614–6.
27. Mazziotti G, Bianchi A, Porcelli T, et al. Vertebral fractures in patients with acromegaly: a 3-year prospective study. J Clin Endocrinol Metab 2013;98:3402–10.
28. Claessen KM, Kroon HM, Pereira AM, et al. Progression of vertebral fractures despite long-term biochemical control of acromegaly: a prospective follow-up study. J Clin Endocrinol Metab 2013;98:4808–15.
29. Giustina A, Casanueva FF, Cavagnini F, et al. Diagnosis and treatment of acromegaly complications. J Endocrinol Invest 2003;26:1242–7.
30. Melmed S, Casanueva FF, Klibanski A, et al. A consensus on the diagnosis and treatment of acromegaly complications. Pituitary 2013;16:294–302.
31. Canalis E, Mazziotti G, Giustina A, et al. Glucocorticoid-induced osteoporosis: pathophysiology and therapy. Osteoporos Int 2007;18:1319–28.
32. Vestergaard P, Lindholm J, Jørgensen JO, et al. Increased risk of osteoporotic fractures in patients with Cushing's syndrome. Eur J Endocrinol 2002;146(1):51–6.
33. Trementino L, Appolloni G, Ceccoli L, et al. Bone complications in patients with Cushing's syndrome: looking for clinical, biochemical, and genetic determinants. Osteoporos Int 2014;25(3):913–21.
34. Scillitani A, Mazziotti G, Di Somma C, et al. Treatment of skeletal impairment in patients with endogenous hypercortisolism: when and how? Osteoporos Int 2014;25(2):441–6.
35. Randazzo ME, Grossrubatscher E, Dalino Ciaramella P, et al. Spontaneous recovery of bone mass after cure of endogenous hypercortisolism. Pituitary 2012;15:193–201.
36. Mancini T, Porcelli T, Giustina A. Treatment of Cushing disease: overview and recent findings. Ther Clin Risk Manag 2010;6:505–16.
37. Di Somma C, Colao A, Pivonello R, et al. Effectiveness of chronic treatment with alendronate in the osteoporosis of Cushing's disease. Clin Endocrinol (Oxf) 1998; 48:655–62.
38. Doga M, Bonadonna S, Gola M, et al. Growth hormone deficiency in the adult. Pituitary 2006;9:305–11.
39. Doga M, Bonadonna S, Gola M, et al. GH deficiency in the adult and bone. J Endocrinol Invest 2005;28(8 Suppl):18–23.
40. Högler W, Shaw N. Childhood growth hormone deficiency, bone density, structures and fractures: scrutinizing the evidence. Clin Endocrinol (Oxf) 2010;72(3):281–9.
41. Murray RD, Adams JE, Shalet SM. A densitometric and morphometric analysis of the skeleton in adults with varying degrees of growth hormone deficiency. J Clin Endocrinol Metab 2006;91(2):432–8.
42. Wuster C, Abs R, Bengtsson BA, et al. The influence of growth hormone deficiency, growth hormone replacement therapy, and other aspects of hypopituitarism on fracture rate and bone mineral density. J Bone Miner Res 2001;16:398–405.
43. Rosen T, Wilhelmsen L, Landin-Wilhelmsen K, et al. Increased fracture frequency in adult patients with hypopituitarism and GH deficiency. Eur J Endocrinol 1997; 137:240–5.
44. Mazziotti G, Bianchi A, Bonadonna S, et al. Increased prevalence of radiological spinal deformities in adult patients with GH deficiency: influence of GH replacement therapy. J Bone Miner Res 2006;21(4):520–8.
45. Mazziotti G, Bianchi A, Cimino V, et al. Effect of gonadal status on bone mineral density and radiological spinal deformities in adult patients with growth hormone deficiency. Pituitary 2008;11:55–61.

46. Ohlsson C, Bengtsson BA, Isaksson OG, et al. Growth hormone and bone. Endocr Rev 1998;19(1):55–79.
47. Barake M, Klibanski A, Tritos NA. Effects of recombinant human growth hormone therapy on bone mineral density in adults with growth hormone deficiency: a meta-analysis. J Clin Endocrinol Metab 2014;99(3):852–60.
48. Hazem A, Elamin MB, Bancos I, et al. Body composition and quality of life in adults treated with GH therapy: a systematic review and meta-analysis. Eur J Endocrinol 2012;166:13–20.
49. Mazziotti G, Mormando M, Cristiano A, et al. Association between l-thyroxine treatment, GH deficiency, and radiological vertebral fractures in patients with adult-onset hypopituitarism. Eur J Endocrinol 2014;170(6):893–9.
50. Mazziotti G, Porcelli T, Bianchi A, et al. Glucocorticoid replacement therapy and vertebral fractures in hypopituitary adult males with GH deficiency. Eur J Endocrinol 2010;163:15–20.

Pituitary Tumor Management in Pregnancy

Paula Bruna Araujo, MD[a], Leonardo Vieira Neto, MD, PhD[a,b],
Mônica R. Gadelha, MD, PhD[a,c],*

KEYWORDS

- Pituitary adenoma • Prolactinomas • Acromegaly • Cushing syndrome
- Cushing disease • TSH-secreting pituitary adenoma
- Nonfunctioning pituitary adenoma • Pregnancy

KEY POINTS

- The general recommendation for pituitary adenoma management is to withdraw medical therapy as soon as pregnancy is diagnosed; however, in cases of aggressive macroadenomas or adenomas close to the optic chiasm, this decision must be individualized according to the patient's status.
- Surgery, when indicated, must be performed during the second trimester of gestation.
- Microadenomas often exhibit a favorable course, and macroadenomas occasionally increase during pregnancy.
- Cushing disease usually leads to a high-risk pregnancy, independent of the size of the pituitary adenoma, because of the deleterious effects of high cortisol levels.
- Close follow-up is the best approach for ensuring the early recognition of complications.

INTRODUCTION

Clinically relevant adenomas have a prevalence of approximately 1 per 1000 in the overall population.[1,2] The adenomas can be functioning or nonfunctioning, and they can impair women's fertility because of the tumor mass and oversecretion of hormones. The improved management of pituitary tumors, either by medical or surgical therapy, has led to an increasing number of pregnancies in patients harboring pituitary adenomas.

The authors have nothing to declare.
[a] Endocrinology Section, Neuroendocrinology Research Center, Medical School and Hospital Universitário Clementino Fraga Filho, Universidade Federal do Rio de Janeiro, Rio de Janeiro, RJ 21941-913, Brazil; [b] Department of Endocrinology, Hospital Federal da Lagoa – Rua Jardim Botânico, 501 Jardim Botânico, Rio de Janeiro, RJ 22470-050, Brazil; [c] Neuroendocrinology Unit, Instituto Estadual do Cérebro – Rua do Rezende, 156 Centro, Rio de Janeiro, RJ 20231-092, Brazil.
* Corresponding author. Hospital Universitário Clementino Fraga Filho, Universidade Federal do Rio de Janeiro, Rua Professor Rodolpho Paulo Rocco, 255, 9° andar, Setor 9F, Sala de Pesquisa em Neuroendocrinolgia, Rio de Janeiro, RJ CEP: 21941-913, Brazil.
E-mail address: mgadelha@hucff.ufrj.br

Pregnancy produces several physiologic changes to the endocrine system, especially to the pituitary gland (**Box 1**). The anterior pituitary gland enlarges by 2-fold to 3-fold during this period,[3] mostly because of hypertrophy and hyperplasia of the lactotrophs stimulated by marked increases in the estrogen levels.[4] Therefore, the endocrinologist faces the challenge of considering the patient's physiologic changes for the effective management of pituitary adenomas during pregnancy to guarantee the wellbeing of the fetus.

PROLACTINOMA

Prolactinomas have an estimated prevalence of 40% of all pituitary adenomas and are primary causes of hyperprolactinemia, which leads to infertility and gonadal dysfunction.[13] Prolactinomas present a peak incidence during childbearing years and are predominantly benign tumors measuring less than 10 mm (microprolactinomas) in more than 90% of cases.[14] Medical therapy with a dopamine agonist (DA) is the first-line treatment and normalizes prolactin levels in 86% of cases,[15] restoring fertility in most patients.[14,16] Transsphenoidal surgery is reserved only for select cases. Thus, pregnancy in these women is a frequent occurrence.

Pregnancy may lead to an increase in prolactinoma size, mainly in pregnant patients with macroprolactinomas.[17] Therefore, these patients should avoid pregnancy by using either hormonal or nonhormonal contraceptive methods until tumor shrinkage occurs.[18] Moreover, women with macroprolactinomas who do not experience pituitary tumor shrinkage during DA therapy or who cannot tolerate DA must be counseled regarding the potential benefits of surgical resection before attempting pregnancy.[16]

Safety of Dopamine Agonists

There are few DAs available for treating these patients; all have been shown to cross the placental barrier.[19] Most studies on pregnancy evaluate bromocriptine and cabergoline, so this article focuses specifically on these.

Box 1
Pituitary gland during normal pregnancy

- Prolactin levels increase up to 10-fold during pregnancy, parallel to the increase in the size of the pituitary gland.[5]

- Although there are hyperplasia and hypertrophy of the lactotrophs, gonadotrophs reduce in number, and corticotrophs and thyrotrophs remain constant.[4]

- The maternal placenta secretes a growth hormone (GH) variant by the end of the first trimester, leading to increased plasma levels of insulinlike growth factor-1 during the second half of pregnancy (up to 2–3 times the upper limit of normal). This leads to somatotroph suppression.[6,7]

- Plasma corticotropin-releasing hormone (CRH) levels (primarily synthesized by the maternal placenta) increase several hundred-fold by term,[8] stimulating the pituitary adrenocorticotropic hormone (ACTH) production.

- The ACTH levels consequently increase throughout gestation, accompanied by increased cortisol levels following the same pattern.[9]

- The increase in total plasma cortisol concentration (up to 2-fold to 3-fold by term) is mostly attributed to a concomitant increase in cortisol-binding globulin (CBG) levels, secondary to estrogen stimulated production.[10]

- The plasma and urinary free cortisol (UFC) start to increase approximately in the 11th week of gestation, incrementing 2 to 3 times during the last 2 trimesters; however, pregnant women normally do not exhibit any overt clinical features of hypercortisolism.[10–12]

It is generally advised to discontinue DA treatment as soon as pregnancy has been confirmed, particularly in patients with microadenomas.[20] When used in this fashion, in more than 6000 pregnancies, bromocriptine has not been found to cause any increase in the incidence of abortion, ectopic pregnancy, trophoblastic disease, or multiple pregnancies, and only 1.8% of the births were affected by congenital malformations, compared with the 3.0% expected in the general population.[21,22]

In recent years, the data concerning cabergoline safety during pregnancy have increased, and more than 800 cases have been published.[23–28] Fetal exposure to cabergoline in early pregnancy seems to be as safe as exposure to bromocriptine (**Table 1**).[23–28] Given the safety profile and the tolerability of cabergoline, this agent has been increasingly used as the first-line therapy in women with prolactinoma who want to become pregnant.[29]

Treatment of Prolactinoma During Pregnancy

The primary goal of prolactinoma treatment during pregnancy is to maintain the adenoma away from the optic chiasm. A review by Molitch[30] pooled information from 514 women with either microadenoma or macroadenoma of any type and showed that only 1.4% of the women with microadenoma presented symptomatic enlargement of the adenoma. Regarding macroadenoma, the behavior of the tumor was more aggressive: 26.2% of the subjects presented symptomatic tumor enlargement. Of the 67 women with macroadenomas with a previous history of surgery or radiation, only 2 women (3%) had symptomatic tumor enlargement.

Therefore, the DA can be safely withdrawn shortly after pregnancy confirmation in patients with microadenoma (**Fig. 1**).[23–28,30,31] These patients should be carefully followed to detect symptoms of tumor enlargement. Visual field testing and MRI (without gadolinium), at any trimester,[32] should be performed only in those cases. This recommendation should be followed for any type of pituitary adenoma that exhibits enlargement during pregnancy.

Because macroprolactinomas have a higher risk of symptomatic tumor enlargement during gestation,[26,30,31] the discontinuation of DA must be individualized, though DA is withdrawn in most patients with intrasellar macroadenomas.[16] In this setting, close surveillance must be performed on a monthly basis. Furthermore, visual field testing is recommended every 2 to 3 months, and MRI is reserved for patients with documented changes in visual field and symptoms of tumor growth.[20,33,34] Maintenance of DA throughout pregnancy may be preferred when previous treatment with DA was administered shortly before conception or when the tumor is located outside of the intrasellar boundaries. Macroprolactinomas with a history of successful surgery or radiation therapy can be managed as microprolactinomas.

If the tumor increase is confirmed for either microadenomas or macroadenomas, treatment should be restarted, more specifically using bromocriptine, according to the published literature.[16] If the enlarged tumor does not respond to DA, alternatives include delivery if the pregnancy is far enough or, during the second trimester, surgical decompression. Periodic evaluation of prolactin levels offers no diagnostic benefit and is not recommended (**Box 2**).[16]

ACROMEGALY

Patients with acromegaly diagnosis frequently have fertility impairment because of the cosecretion of prolactin and the mass effects of the tumor affecting the gonadotrophic axis.[37] Nevertheless, pregnancy among acromegalic patients is becoming more common due to improvements in treatment as well as in fertility therapies.

Table 1
Summary of the series reported about cabergoline use during pregnancy in subjects harboring a prolactinoma

Series	Number of Subjects/ Pregnancies	Sellar Images (Available)	Time of Exposition	Dose Range (Per Week)	Maternal Complications (Number of Cases)	Gestational Outcomes	Deliveries (Known Duration)	Fetal Outcomes
Robert et al,[23] 1996	205/226	118 Microadenomas 15 Macroadenomas 5 Empty sella 65 Normal (ID)	1 to 144 d	0.125–4.0 mg	None	23 Spontaneous abortions 31 Terminations (3 for malformation) 1 IUFD 1 Ectopic pregnancy	129 Term 17 Premature 2 Missing data All single births	148 Live births (10 SGA and 10 LGA) 7 Malformations (3.1%) (2 major) 22 Unknown
Ricci et al,[24] 2002	50/61	25 Microadenomas 12 Macroadenomas 2 Empty sella 5 Normal (ID)	7 to 266 d (mean 39.3 d)	0.25–7.0 mg (mean dose 1.1 mg)	None	6 Spontaneous abortions 5 Terminations (1 for malformation) 1 Hydatidiform moles	38 Term 3 Premature 8 Missing data All single births	49 Live births (6 SGA) 2 Malformation (3.3%) (1 major)
Colao et al,[25] 2008	329/329	N/A	<1 mo in 33% 1–2 mo in 47%	Mean dose 0.98 mg	N/A	31 Spontaneous abortions 40 Terminations (9 for malformation)	193 Term 45 Premature 12 Unknown (8 twin)	250 Live births (17 SGA and 9 LGA) 23 Malformations (6.9%) 4 Stillbirths 4 Unknown
Lebbe et al,[26] 2010	72/100	45 Microadenomas 15 Macroadenomas 12 Normal (ID)	7 to 154 d (median 28 d)	0.25–1.5 mg (median dose 0.5 mg)	3 Hypertension 1 Preeclampsia 4 Gestational diabetes	10 Spontaneous abortions 5 Terminations (3 malformations; 1 twin)	76 Term 8 Premature (4 twin)	88 Live births (9 SGA) 3 Malformations (3.0%) (All major)

						termination) 2 Ectopic pregnancies		
Ono et al,[27] 2010	80/93	53 Microadenomas 27 Macroadenomas	<4 wk in all pregnancies	Maximum dose of 3.0 mg (mean dose 2.29 mg)	1 Hypertension	1 Spontaneous abortion 1 Termination 1 IUFD	82 Term 1 Premature All single births	83 Live births (9 SGA) 7 Ongoing pregnancies No malformations
Auriemma et al,[28] 2013	91/143	76 Microadenomas 10 Macroadenomas 5 Normal (ID)	<6 wk in all pregnancies	(Mean dose 0.69 mg)	None	13 Spontaneous abortions 4 Terminations (1 therapeutic)	126 Term 0 Premature All single births	126 Live births (2 SGA) No malformations
Total	827/952	317 Microadenomas 79 Macroadenomas 7 Empty sella 87 Normal (ID)	N/A	N/A	4 Hypertension 1 Preeclampsia 4 Gestational diabetes	83 Spontaneous abortions 86 Terminations 6 IUFDs 3 Ectopic pregnancies 1 Hydatidiform mole 4 Unknown status	644 Term 74 Premature	744 Live births 35 Malformations (3.7%)

Abbreviations: ID, idiopathic disease; IUFD, intrauterine fetal death; LGA, large for gestational age; SGA, small for gestational age.
Data from Refs.[23–28]

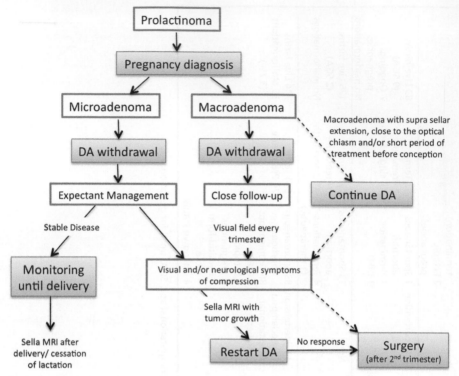

Fig. 1. Prolactinoma management during pregnancy. DA, dopamine agonist.

Box 2
Lactation and follow-up after delivery for women with prolactinoma

- Women who wish to breastfeed their infants should not be given DA because the resulting decrease in serum prolactin levels will impair lactation.[14]

- Patients who must receive DA to prevent tumor growth should continue their treatment, although lactation will be impaired.

- No data suggest that breastfeeding leads to an increase in tumor size. Furthermore, prolactin levels are often lower than before pregnancy.

- The recent studies by Domingue and colleagues[35] and Auriemma and colleagues[28] showed that 41% and 68% of women with prolactinoma, respectively, were in remission of hyperprolactinemia after pregnancy and lactation at a median time interval of 22 months and up to 60 months, respectively. In both studies, breastfeeding did not increase the risk of recurrence of hyperprolactinemia.

- Patients should be reassessed 2 months after delivery or after cessation of lactation, and a pituitary imaging is recommended to evaluate the adenoma.[29]

- If MRI is necessary during lactation, it can be performed using gadolinium. Less than 1% of this contrast is excreted into the breast milk.[36] Therefore, the decision to continue or to suspend breastfeeding for 24 h after a scan should be determined by the doctor and the mother.[36]

The occurrence of pregnancy associated with acromegaly is concerning because the risk of complications, such as gestational diabetes and hypertension, are increased, especially in women with growth hormone (GH) or insulinlike growth factor-1 (IGF-1) not controlled before conception.[38] Regarding the fetus, limited publications have reported normal full-term infants in most cases, with a few cases of low birth weight, which is often related to treatment using somatostatin analogue (SA).[38–40]

No tumor enlargement was diagnosed in subjects with prior surgery and/or radio-therapy of macroadenomas in series of acromegalic pregnant subjects.[39–42] However, in the presence of a high Ki-67 labeling index and low aryl hydrocarbon receptor-interacting protein expression, tumor enlargement may occur during gestation even after transsphenoidal surgery.[43] Most women with untreated acromegaly have uneventful pregnancies, especially those with microadenomas; however, several subjects required transsphenoidal surgery for pituitary apoplexy associated with GH-secreting macroadenomas or advancing visual loss (**Box 3**).[38,42]

Treatment of Acromegaly During Pregnancy

Among the medications available for treating acromegaly, SAs are more efficacious than DAs[50,51]; however, SAs have not been used frequently during pregnancy. Women planning to get pregnant should discontinue medical therapy with a long-acting SA 2 to 3 months before conception, depending on their clinical status.[46,52]

In several recent series,[38–41] pregnant women with acromegaly received SA during pregnancy, sometimes with concomitant DA; however, in most cases, the medication was stopped as soon as gestation was diagnosed. Even considering cases in which there was prolonged use of SA during gestation, no serious adverse events regarding pregnancy, delivery, and newborn development were observed (**Table 2**).[38–41,53] The GH-receptor antagonist use is restricted to exceptional case reports of uncomplicated pregnancies in acromegalic subjects.[54,55]

Box 3
Pregnancy and acromegaly

- In pregnant acromegalic women, the secretion of placental GH induces an increase in plasma IGF-1 level but not a decrease in the autonomous secretion of GH by the pituitary adenoma.[44]

- To diagnose acromegaly in pregnancy, an interference-free immunofluorometric assay specific for placental GH variant is required to differentiate the pituitary GH and the placental GH.[45]

- The presence of both maternal GH and placental GH in the maternal blood, along with elevated IGF-1, makes it difficult to definitively diagnose acromegaly during gestation. Therefore, biochemical monitoring is of limited use.[46]

- Despite additional placenta-derived GH during pregnancy, acromegalic patients often report an improvement in their clinical signs and symptoms, especially during the first trimester of pregnancy.

- A reduction in IGF-1 levels during pregnancy of acromegalic patients is often noted even without medical therapy,[38–41,47] whereas a variable decrease in pituitary GH concentrations has been reported in the second half of pregnancy.[48]

- The improvement in IGF-1 could be attributed to the effect of the marked increase in estrogen levels during pregnancy, which inhibits GH signaling, an action that is mediated by the suppressor of cytokine signaling (SOCS) proteins, resulting in a state of GH resistance.[47,49]

Table 2
Summary of the series reported about acromegaly during pregnancy with use of somatostatin analogue

Series	Number of Subjects/ Pregnancies	Adenoma Size (Available)	Time of Diagnosis	Nonmedical Treatment Before Pregnancy	Treatment During Pregnancy	Acromegaly Course During Pregnancy	Maternal Complications or Gestational Outcome	Fetal Outcome
Cozzi et al,[41] 2006	6/7	4 Macro 2 Micro	All subjects diagnosed before pregnancy	3 Neurosurgeries 1 Neurosurgery and radiotherapy	2 Subjects discontinued depot SA after confirmation of pregnancy Others stopped medication 3–4 mo before conception (DA and/or SA)	GH status: increased in 11, stable in 3, and decreased in 3 subjects IGF-1 status: stable, close to normal range in all subjects 1 Subject refused surgery before pregnancy and was on depot SA, presented tumor enlargement, but no visual field	No complications 7 Term pregnancies	7 Live births, all normal newborns
Caron et al,[38] 2010	46/59	39 Macro 7 Micro	6 Subjects had acromegaly diagnosis during pregnancy	39 Neurosurgeries 9 Conventional radiotherapies 5 Gamma-knife radiotherapies	25 Subjects conceived using DA treatment and 14 subjects conceived using SA treatment (8 used both drugs) In most cases, medical treatment discontinued when pregnancy was diagnosed	GH status: mean values were stable IGF-1 status: significant reduction during the 1st and 2nd trimesters 4 Cases of visual field defect (leading to diagnosis of acromegaly in 3 cases, 1 submitted to neurosurgery at 2nd trimester)	4 Cases of GD, 4 cases of hypertension, 1 case of preeclampsia 2 Spontaneous abortions 2 Terminations 55 Term 4 Premature 5 Twin	64 Live births (6 SGA and 2 LGA) No malformations

Cheng et al,[39] 2012	12/13	5 Macro 3 Micro 4 N/A	All subjects diagnosed before pregnancy	6 Neurosurgeries	3 Subjects conceived using SA treatment 1 Case, SA used during 1st trimester 2 Cases, SA used for 20 wk of gestation	IGF-1 status: remained stable or decreased	No complications 13 Term pregnancies	13 Live births (1 SGA, from a subject treated during pregnancy) No malformations
Dias et al,[40] 2014	8/10	8 Macro	All subjects were diagnosed before pregnancy	8 Neurosurgeries	9 Pregnancies started with SA treatment 4 Pregnancies started with SA and DA treatment Pharmacologic treatment withdrawn at pregnancy diagnosed (5–6 wk)	GH status: levels assessed in 5 subjects with no significant changes (significant decline in GH was observed in normal pregnant controls) IGF-1 status: mean levels remained unchanged, although the range has increased significantly after midgestation	3 Cases headache, 1 case of GDM and 1 case of hypertension, followed by preeclampsia 9 Term 1 Premature	10 Live births (1 SGA, from subject with preeclampsia) No malformations

Abbreviations: GH, growth hormone; IGF-1, insulinlike growth factor-1; LGA, large for gestational age; SGA, small for gestational age.
Data from Refs.[38–41]

Nevertheless, a clinical approach to pregnant acromegalic patients is usually expectant, and the withdrawal of any medical therapy for acromegaly treatment is recommended in most cases, along with close follow-up during gestation (**Fig. 2**).[46,52]

In patients with GH-secreting macroadenomas, although tumor enlargement rarely occurs,[38–41] close follow-up and visual field testing are recommended every trimester, independent of the development of compressive symptoms and with the use of MRI limited to confirming tumor enlargement.[46,52] For patients with a macroadenoma diagnosed during pregnancy or after a short medical treatment (less than 1 year), monthly follow-up visits should be proposed.[52] Patients with macroadenomas at high risk for tumor growth can be maintained on treatment with DA and/or SA throughout the pregnancy.[43,46,53] In patients with evidence of tumor growth, transsphenoidal surgery during the second trimester and/or medical treatment should be considered, and breastfeeding is contraindicated.[34,52]

There are only 2 reports of transsphenoidal surgery in acromegalic pregnant patients.[56,57] In both cases, the diagnosis of acromegaly was made at the last trimester due to visual complaints: 1 patient had acute visual loss and the other had pituitary apoplexy. Both underwent emergent transsphenoidal surgery. One patient delivered at term, whereas the other patient had a cesarean section at 34 weeks. Both babies were healthy.

In uneventful pregnancies, breastfeeding is allowed before the commencement of pharmacologic treatment because of the lack of complications documented in

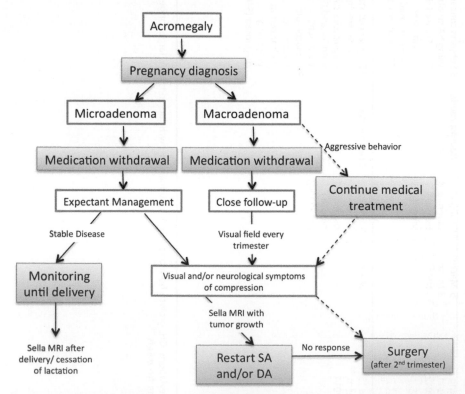

Fig. 2. Acromegaly management during pregnancy. DA, dopamine agonist; SA, somatostatin analogues.

lactating women with acromegaly.[38–41] After delivery, MRI must be repeated in all patients with GH-secreting tumors to evaluate the tumor size.[34]

CUSHING SYNDROME

Pregnancy rarely occurs during the course of Cushing syndrome (CS) because the disease leads to a state of hypercortisolism and hyperandrogenism that suppress the gonadotroph function. This condition results in oligomenorrhea and amenorrhea in most female patients, frequently accompanied by infertility.[58]

Different from cases of prolactinoma and acromegaly, in which the disease is usually diagnosed before pregnancy, CS was diagnosed during the course of pregnancy in most reported cases.[59] An adrenal adenoma is responsible for most of these cases, with only 40% related to an adrenocorticotropic hormone (ACTH)-producing pituitary adenoma.[29]

Cushing Syndrome Diagnosis and Differential Diagnosis During Pregnancy

The clinical diagnosis of CS during pregnancy may be missed because of the overlapping features of weight gain, hypertension, fatigue, hyperglycemia, and emotional changes characteristic of pregnancy.[60] Clues that can lead to suspicion of CS include large purple instead of white striae, hirsutism, acne, the presence of hypokalemia, muscle weakness, and pathologic fractures.[61,62]

The diagnostic tests for CS become less reliable during gestation (**Box 4**), and the normal physiology of pregnancy makes it difficult to biochemically diagnose CS (see **Box 1**). The differential diagnosis among all possible causes of CS is mandatory to address the therapeutic approach. Therefore, plasma ACTH measurement should be the initial step to guide the subsequent evaluation with pituitary or adrenal MRI.[59]

Treatment of Cushing Syndrome During Pregnancy

The association of pregnancy with CS increases maternal morbidity in approximately 70% of cases and also impairs fetal outcome (**Table 3**).[11,29] Therefore, there is a rationale for treating CS during pregnancy. However, treating pregnant patients with CS has been done only sporadically, generally late in the course of the pregnancy.

Box 4
Establishing Cushing syndrome diagnosis during gestation

- Low-dose dexamethasone administration usually fails to suppress cortisol secretion during pregnancy.[29] According to the guidelines for diagnosis of CS, the use of this test during pregnancy should not be preferred because of false-positive results due to blunted response to dexamethasone.[63]

- Another problem is that plasma cortisol will be elevated because of an increase in CBG.[64]

- UFC should be used as the best choice in screening for CS during pregnancy. Values greater than 3 times the upper limit should be taken into consideration in the last 2 trimesters.[63]

- Because serum cortisol circadian variation is altered in women with CS but preserved in normal pregnancy, late-night cortisol greater than 5 mg/dL or greater than 50% of morning cortisol is suggestive of CS.[11]

- Nighttime salivary cortisol measurement is the best test to evaluate the circadian rhythm of cortisol and theoretically could be a good screening test for CS during pregnancy, although there is no specific study that defines the cutoff during gestation.[65,66]

Table 3
Maternal and fetal complications in Cushing syndrome during pregnancy

Maternal Morbidity	Fetal Morbidity
Hypertension	Spontaneous abortion or intrauterine death
Diabetes mellitus	Prematurity
Preeclampsia	Stillbirth
Osteoporosis and fracture	Intrauterine growth retardation
Cardiac failure	Infant death
Pulmonary edema	Hypoadrenalism
Psychiatric disorder	Intraventricular hemorrhage postpartum
Wound infection	Malformation
Maternal death	—

Consequently, the ability of treatment to prevent adverse outcomes is not well-established,[60] although a trend toward better fetal outcome in treated patients compared with nontreated patients has been observed.[59]

Concerning ACTH-secreting adenomas, which is the scope of this article, the treatment of choice is transsphenoidal surgery during the second trimester of pregnancy.[29,67] Despite that recommendation, among all cases of CS reported in a review by Lindsay and colleagues,[59] only 20% of the patients underwent transsphenoidal surgery; the remainder of the treated patients received medical therapy (metyrapone or ketoconazole) and/or adrenalectomy. A high proportion (54%) of the patients was untreated.

In cases in which surgery cannot be performed, such as severe CS, medical treatment can be considered. The primary medical therapy was reported in 20 women, most using metyrapone, which seems to be well tolerated although it is occasionally associated with preeclampsia. Therefore, its use must be limited to a transient period, pending a definitive approach.[59] Ketoconazole has been successfully used in 3 pregnancies without adverse events.[59] However, because of its antiandrogenic effects and teratogenicity demonstrated in rats, this medication should be reserved for individuals who need emergent medical therapy and who cannot tolerate metyrapone.[59] A recent case report concerning the use of cabergoline in high doses throughout pregnancy showed a favorable outcome, suggesting a possible role for DA in the treatment of pregnant patients with CS.[68]

THYROTROPIN PITUITARY ADENOMAS

Thyrotropin is also called thyroid-secreting hormone (TSH). TSH pituitary adenomas (TSH-omas) account for approximately 0.5% to 3% of all pituitary adenomas.[69] They are often large and invasive lesions associated with symptoms of hyperthyroidism.[69] Pregnancy in women harboring TSH-omas is, therefore, exceedingly rare, with only 4 cases reported in the literature. The pituitary adenoma diagnosis occurred before pregnancy in 3 cases and during pregnancy in 1 case, all of which resulted in healthy newborns.[70–73]

As with other pituitary adenomas, patients with TSH-omas require close follow-up for mass-related tumor symptoms. Because this adenoma subtype is rare, a general management strategy cannot be established. Nevertheless, successful outcomes from previously reported cases demonstrate that pregnancy is feasible in these patients.

NONFUNCTIONING PITUITARY ADENOMAS

Nonfunctioning pituitary adenomas (NFPAs) represent approximately 30% of all pituitary tumors.[74] They are usually diagnosed at the sixth decade, being rare in women of reproductive age.[75] Because fertility is usually impaired due to hypopituitarism, pregnancy rarely occurs in women with NFPAs.

Pregnancy rarely increases the size of clinical NFPAs. The enlargement of the pituitary adenoma may be due to tumor growth or apoplexy of the tumor during pregnancy.[29] The best approach for patients with asymptomatic NFPA is the wait-and-see policy. However, in cases of symptomatic tumor enlargement, medical treatment using DA can be considered to reduce physiologic lactotroph cell hyperplasia, and surgery should be considered during the second trimester.[29,34]

SUMMARY

The general recommendation for pituitary adenoma patients is to withdraw medical therapy as soon as pregnancy is diagnosed. However, in cases of macroadenomas, this decision must be individualized. Moreover, when medical therapy is imperative, commonly used medications (eg, DA and SA) seem to be safe. Surgery, when indicated, must be performed during the second trimester of gestation. Those recommendations are not applicable to pregnant women with CS in which there is a high risk of complications for both mother and fetus, independent of the pituitary adenoma size, due to the deleterious effects of high cortisol levels. In this setting, either medical or surgical treatment can be considered during pregnancy.

Available data show that microadenomas often exhibit a favorable course and that macroadenomas occasionally increase in size. A concern regarding visual compression exists primarily because the pituitary gland suffers an estrogen-induced lactotroph hyperplasia; however, this physiologic phenomenon is usually not enough to lead to compressive symptoms, unless the tumor itself suffers an enlargement. Nevertheless, close follow-up is the best approach for ensuring early recognition of complications.

REFERENCES

1. Daly AF, Rixhon M, Adam C, et al. High prevalence of pituitary adenomas: a cross-sectional study in the province of Liege, Belgium. J Clin Endocrinol Metab 2006;91(12):4769–75.
2. Fernandez A, Karavitaki N, Wass JA. Prevalence of pituitary adenomas: a community-based, cross-sectional study in Banbury (Oxfordshire, UK). Clin Endocrinol 2010;72(3):377–82.
3. Gonzalez JG, Elizondo G, Saldivar D, et al. Pituitary gland growth during normal pregnancy: an in vivo study using magnetic resonance imaging. Am J Med 1988; 85(2):217–20.
4. Scheithauer BW, Sano T, Kovacs KT, et al. The pituitary gland in pregnancy: a clinicopathologic and immunohistochemical study of 69 cases. Mayo Clin Proc 1990;65(4):461–74.
5. Rigg LA, Lein A, Yen SS. Pattern of increase in circulating prolactin levels during human gestation. Am J Obstet Gynecol 1977;129(4):454–6.
6. Caufriez A, Frankenne F, Hennen G, et al. Regulation of maternal IGF-I by placental GH in normal and abnormal human pregnancies. Am J Physiol 1993; 265(4 Pt 1):E572–7.

7. Frankenne F, Closset J, Gomez F, et al. The physiology of growth hormones (GHs) in pregnant women and partial characterization of the placental GH variant. J Clin Endocrinol Metab 1988;66(6):1171–80.

8. Stalla GK, Bost H, Stalla J, et al. Human corticotropin-releasing hormone during pregnancy. Gynecol Endocrinol 1989;3(1):1–10.

9. Sasaki A, Shinkawa O, Yoshinaga K. Placental corticotropin-releasing hormone may be a stimulator of maternal pituitary adrenocorticotropic hormone secretion in humans. J Clin Invest 1989;84(6):1997–2001.

10. Nolten WE, Lindheimer MD, Rueckert PA, et al. Diurnal patterns and regulation of cortisol secretion in pregnancy. J Clin Endocrinol Metab 1980;51(3):466–72.

11. Lindsay JR, Nieman LK. The hypothalamic-pituitary-adrenal axis in pregnancy: challenges in disease detection and treatment. Endocr Rev 2005;26(6): 775–99.

12. Feldt-Rasmussen U, Mathiesen ER. Endocrine disorders in pregnancy: physiological and hormonal aspects of pregnancy. Best Pract Res Clin Endocrinol Metab 2011;25(6):875–84.

13. Schlechte JA. Clinical practice. Prolactinoma. N Engl J Med 2003;349(21): 2035–41.

14. Casanueva FF, Molitch ME, Schlechte JA, et al. Guidelines of the Pituitary Society for the diagnosis and management of prolactinomas. Clin Endocrinol 2006;65(2): 265–73.

15. Verhelst J, Abs R, Maiter D, et al. Cabergoline in the treatment of hyperprolactinemia: a study in 455 patients. J Clin Endocrinol Metab 1999;84(7): 2518–22.

16. Melmed S, Casanueva FF, Hoffman AR, et al. Diagnosis and treatment of hyperprolactinemia: an Endocrine Society clinical practice guideline. J Clin Endocrinol Metab 2011;96(2):273–88.

17. Molitch ME. Pregnancy and the hyperprolactinemic woman. N Engl J Med 1985; 312(21):1364–70.

18. Moraes AB, Silva CM, Vieira Neto L, et al. Giant prolactinomas: the therapeutic approach. Clin Endocrinol 2013;79(4):447–56.

19. Kars M, Dekkers OM, Pereira AM, et al. Update in prolactinomas. Neth J Med 2010;68(3):104–12.

20. Molitch ME. Prolactinoma in pregnancy. Best Pract Res Clin Endocrinol Metab 2011;25(6):885–96.

21. Molitch ME. Prolactinomas and pregnancy. Clin Endocrinol 2010;73(2):147–8.

22. Krupp P, Monka C. Bromocriptine in pregnancy: safety aspects. Klin Wochenschr 1987;65(17):823–7.

23. Robert E, Musatti L, Piscitelli G, et al. Pregnancy outcome after treatment with the ergot derivative, cabergoline. Reprod Toxicol 1996;10(4):333–7.

24. Ricci E, Parazzini F, Motta T, et al. Pregnancy outcome after cabergoline treatment in early weeks of gestation. Reprod Toxicol 2002;16(6):791–3.

25. Colao A, Abs R, Barcena DG, et al. Pregnancy outcomes following cabergoline treatment: extended results from a 12-year observational study. Clin Endocrinol 2008;68(1):66–71.

26. Lebbe M, Hubinont C, Bernard P, et al. Outcome of 100 pregnancies initiated under treatment with cabergoline in hyperprolactinaemic women. Clin Endocrinol 2010;73(2):236–42.

27. Ono M, Miki N, Amano K, et al. Individualized high-dose cabergoline therapy for hyperprolactinemic infertility in women with micro- and macroprolactinomas. J Clin Endocrinol Metab 2010;95(6):2672–9.

28. Auriemma RS, Perone Y, Di Sarno A, et al. Results of a single-center observational 10-year survey study on recurrence of hyperprolactinemia after pregnancy and lactation. J Clin Endocrinol Metab 2013;98(1):372–9.
29. Karaca Z, Tanriverdi F, Unluhizarci K, et al. Pregnancy and pituitary disorders. Eur J Endocrinol 2010;162(3):453–75.
30. Molitch ME. Pituitary tumors and pregnancy. Growth Horm IGF Res 2003; 13(Suppl A):S38–44.
31. Bronstein MD. Prolactinomas and pregnancy. Pituitary 2005;8(1):31–8.
32. Kanal E, Barkovich AJ, Bell C, et al. ACR guidance document on MR safe practices: 2013. J Magn Reson Imaging 2013;37(3):501–30.
33. Karaca Z, Kelestimur F. Pregnancy and other pituitary disorders (including GH deficiency). Best Pract Res Clin Endocrinol Metab 2011;25(6):897–910.
34. Pivonello R, De Martino MC, Auriemma RS, et al. Pituitary tumors and pregnancy: the interplay between a pathologic condition and a physiologic status. J Endocrinol Invest 2014;37(2):99–112.
35. Domingue ME, Devuyst F, Alexopoulou O, et al. Outcome of prolactinoma after pregnancy and lactation: a study on 73 patients. Clin Endocrinol 2014;80(5):642–8.
36. Cova MA, Stacul F, Quaranta R, et al. Radiological contrast media in the breastfeeding woman: a position paper of the Italian Society of Radiology (SIRM), the Italian Society of Paediatrics (SIP), the Italian Society of Neonatology (SIN) and the Task Force on Breastfeeding, Ministry of Health, Italy. Eur Radiol 2014;24:2012–22.
37. Grynberg M, Salenave S, Young J, et al. Female gonadal function before and after treatment of acromegaly. J Clin Endocrinol Metab 2010;95(10):4518–25.
38. Caron P, Broussaud S, Bertherat J, et al. Acromegaly and pregnancy: a retrospective multicenter study of 59 pregnancies in 46 women. J Clin Endocrinol Metab 2010;95(10):4680–7.
39. Cheng S, Grasso L, Martinez-Orozco JA, et al. Pregnancy in acromegaly: experience from two referral centers and systematic review of the literature. Clin Endocrinol 2012;76(2):264–71.
40. Dias M, Boguszewski C, Gadelha M, et al. Acromegaly and pregnancy: a prospective study. Eur J Endocrinol 2014;170(2):301–10.
41. Cozzi R, Attanasio R, Barausse M. Pregnancy in acromegaly: a one-center experience. Eur J Endocrinol 2006;155(2):279–84.
42. Atmaca A, Dagdelen S, Erbas T. Follow-up of pregnancy in acromegalic women: different presentations and outcomes. Exp Clin Endocrinol Diabetes 2006;114(3): 135–9.
43. Kasuki L, Neto LV, Takiya CM, et al. Growth of an aggressive tumor during pregnancy in an acromegalic patient. Endocr J 2012;59(4):313–9.
44. Beckers A, Stevenaert A, Foidart JM, et al. Placental and pituitary growth hormone secretion during pregnancy in acromegalic women. J Clin Endocrinol Metab 1990;71(3):725–31.
45. Dias ML, Vieira JG, Abucham J. Detecting and solving the interference of pregnancy serum, in a GH immunometric assay. Growth Horm IGF Res 2013; 23(1–2):13–8.
46. Katznelson L, Atkinson JL, Cook DM, et al. American Association of Clinical Endocrinologists medical guidelines for clinical practice for the diagnosis and treatment of acromegaly–2011 update. Endocr Pract 2011;17(Suppl 4):1–44.
47. Lau SL, McGrath S, Evain-Brion D, et al. Clinical and biochemical improvement in acromegaly during pregnancy. J Endocrinol Invest 2008;31(3):255–61.
48. Wiesli P, Zwimpfer C, Zapf J, et al. Pregnancy-induced changes in insulin-like growth factor I (IGF-I), insulin-like growth factor binding protein 3 (IGFBP-3), and

acid-labile subunit (ALS) in patients with growth hormone (GH) deficiency and excess. Acta Obstet Gynecol Scand 2006;85(8):900–5.

49. Leung KC, Johannsson G, Leong GM, et al. Estrogen regulation of growth hormone action. Endocr Rev 2004;25(5):693–721.

50. Colao A, Ferone D, Marzullo P, et al. Effect of different dopaminergic agents in the treatment of acromegaly. J Clin Endocrinol Metab 1997;82(2):518–23.

51. Vieira Neto L, Abucham J, Araujo LA, et al. Recommendations of Neuroendocrinology Department from Brazilian Society of Endocrinology and Metabolism for diagnosis and treatment of acromegaly in Brazil. Arq Bras Endocrinol Metabol 2011;55(9):725–6.

52. Caron P. Acromegaly and pregnancy. Ann Endocrinol (Paris) 2011;72(4): 282–6.

53. Maffei P, Tamagno G, Nardelli GB, et al. Effects of octreotide exposure during pregnancy in acromegaly. Clin Endocrinol 2010;72(5):668–77.

54. Qureshi A, Kalu E, Ramanathan G, et al. IVF/ICSI in a woman with active acromegaly: successful outcome following treatment with pegvisomant. J Assist Reprod Genet 2006;23(11–12):439–42.

55. Brian SR, Bidlingmaier M, Wajnrajch MP, et al. Treatment of acromegaly with pegvisomant during pregnancy: maternal and fetal effects. J Clin Endocrinol Metab 2007;92(9):3374–7.

56. Lunardi P, Rizzo A, Missori P, et al. Pituitary apoplexy in an acromegalic woman operated on during pregnancy by transphenoidal approach. Int J Gynaecol Obstet 1991;34(1):71–4.

57. Guven S, Durukan T, Berker M, et al. A case of acromegaly in pregnancy: concomitant transsphenoidal adenomectomy and cesarean section. J Matern Fetal Neonatal Med 2006;19(1):69–71.

58. Bertagna X, Guignat L, Groussin L, et al. Cushing's disease. Best Pract Res Clin Endocrinol Metab 2009;23(5):607–23.

59. Lindsay JR, Jonklaas J, Oldfield EH, et al. Cushing's syndrome during pregnancy: personal experience and review of the literature. J Clin Endocrinol Metab 2005;90(5):3077–83.

60. Vilar L, Freitas Mda C, Lima LH, et al. Cushing's syndrome in pregnancy: an overview. Arq Bras Endocrinol Metabol 2007;51(8):1293–302.

61. Prebtani AP, Donat D, Ezzat S. Worrisome striae in pregnancy. Lancet 2000; 355(9216):1692.

62. Tajika T, Shinozaki T, Watanabe H, et al. Case report of a Cushing's syndrome patient with multiple pathologic fractures during pregnancy. J Orthop Sci 2002; 7(4):498–500.

63. Nieman LK, Biller BM, Findling JW, et al. The diagnosis of Cushing's syndrome: an Endocrine Society Clinical Practice Guideline. J Clin Endocrinol Metab 2008; 93(5):1526–40.

64. Scott EM, McGarrigle HH, Lachelin GC. The increase in plasma and saliva cortisol levels in pregnancy is not due to the increase in corticosteroid-binding globulin levels. J Clin Endocrinol Metab 1990;71(3):639–44.

65. Viardot A, Huber P, Puder JJ, et al. Reproducibility of nighttime salivary cortisol and its use in the diagnosis of hypercortisolism compared with urinary free cortisol and overnight dexamethasone suppression test. J Clin Endocrinol Metab 2005;90(10):5730–6.

66. Manetti L, Rossi G, Grasso L, et al. Usefulness of salivary cortisol in the diagnosis of hypercortisolism: comparison with serum and urinary cortisol. Eur J Endocrinol 2013;168(3):315–21.

67. Mellor A, Harvey RD, Pobereskin LH, et al. Cushing's disease treated by trans-sphenoidal selective adenomectomy in mid-pregnancy. Br J Anaesth 1998; 80(6):850–2.

68. Woo I, Ehsanipoor RM. Cabergoline therapy for Cushing disease throughout pregnancy. Obstet Gynecol 2013;122(2 Pt 2):485–7.

69. Beck-Peccoz P, Lania A, Beckers A, et al. 2013 European thyroid association guidelines for the diagnosis and treatment of thyrotropin-secreting pituitary tumors. Eur Thyroid J 2013;2(2):76–82.

70. Caron P, Gerbeau C, Pradayrol L, et al. Successful pregnancy in an infertile woman with a thyrotropin-secreting macroadenoma treated with somatostatin analog (octreotide). J Clin Endocrinol Metab 1996;81(3):1164–8.

71. Chaiamnuay S, Moster M, Katz MR, et al. Successful management of a pregnant woman with a TSH secreting pituitary adenoma with surgical and medical therapy. Pituitary 2003;6(2):109–13.

72. Blackhurst G, Strachan MW, Collie D, et al. The treatment of a thyrotropin-secreting pituitary macroadenoma with octreotide in twin pregnancy. Clin Endocrinol 2002; 57(3):401–4.

73. Bolz M, Korber S, Schober HC. TSH secreting adenoma of pituitary gland (TSHom) - rare cause of hyperthyroidism in pregnancy. Dtsch Med Wochenschr 2013;138(8):362–6.

74. Jaffe CA. Clinically non-functioning pituitary adenoma. Pituitary 2006;9(4): 317–21.

75. Greenman Y, Stern N. Non-functioning pituitary adenomas. Best Pract Res Clin Endocrinol Metab 2009;23(5):625–38.

Pituitary Apoplexy

Claire Briet, MD, PhD[a,b], Sylvie Salenave, MD[a],
Philippe Chanson, MD[a,b,c],*

KEYWORDS

- Pituitary apoplexy • Emergency • Neurosurgery • Magnetic resonance imaging
- Hemorrhage • Necrosis • Pituitary adenoma • Corticotropic deficiency

KEY POINTS

- Pituitary apoplexy is caused by sudden hemorrhaging or infarction of the pituitary gland, generally within an undiagnosed pituitary adenoma.
- Headache of sudden and severe onset is the main symptom, associated with visual disturbances or ocular palsy in half the cases.
- Corticotropic deficiency may be life-threatening if untreated.
- Computed tomography (CT) or MRI confirms the diagnosis by revealing a pituitary tumor with hemorrhagic and/or necrotic components: CT is most useful in the acute setting (24–48 h), whereas MRI is useful for identifying blood components in the subacute setting (4 days–1 month).
- As the course of pituitary apoplexy is highly variable, optimal management is controversial: some investigators advocate early transphenoidal surgical decompression, whereas others adopt a more conservative approach for selected patients, especially those without visual defects and with normal consciousness.
- Glucocorticoid treatment must always be started immediately, as it may be life-saving.

INTRODUCTION

Pituitary apoplexy (PA) is an acute clinical syndrome caused by sudden hemorrhaging and/or infarction of the pituitary gland, generally within a pituitary adenoma. The outcome of acute apoplexy within a pituitary adenoma is difficult to predict: the patient's clinical condition may deteriorate dramatically (subarachnoid hemorrhage from an apoplectic adenoma or cerebral ischemia secondary to cerebral vasospasm), or improve spontaneously, with or without sequelae, such as visual defects, neurologic disorders, and pituitary insufficiency. Apoplexy sometimes destroys the pituitary adenoma but regrowth from a tumor remnant may occur in other cases.

The authors have no conflicts of interest to disclose.

[a] Assistance Publique-Hôpitaux de Paris, Hôpital de Bicêtre, Department of Endocrinology and Reproductive Diseases, Le Kremlin-Bicêtre F-94275, France; [b] Univ Paris-Sud, School of Medicine, Orsay F-91405, France; [c] Insitut National de la Santé et de la Recherche Médicale, Unit 693, Le Kremlin-Bicêtre, F-94276, France
* Corresponding author. Department of Endocrinology and Reproductive Diseases, Hôpital de Bicêtre, 78 rue du Général Leclerc, Le Kremlin-Bicêtre 94275, France.
E-mail address: philippe.chanson@bct.aphp.fr

EPIDEMIOLOGY, PREDISPOSING FACTORS, AND PRECIPITATING FACTORS

PA has a prevalence of 6.2 cases per 100,000 inhabitants[1] and an incidence of 0.17 episodes per 100,000 person-years.[2] Apoplexy, which occurs in 2% to 12% of patients with all types of adenoma[3–8] (preferentially nonfunctioning pituitary adenomas [NFPA][1,3,5,9–11]), is the first manifestation in 80% of them.[3] The risk of PA is low (0.2–0.6 events per 100 person-years) in patients with conservatively managed NFPA or incidentalomas.[12,13]

PA can occur at all ages but is most frequent in the fifth or sixth decade and shows a slight male preponderance.

Precipitating factors are identified in 20% to 40% of cases.[3,5,6,9–11,14–16] An acute increase in intracranial pressure, arterial hypertension, angiographic procedures, and major surgery (particularly cardiac surgery, because of blood pressure fluctuations and anticoagulant therapy) are well-known triggers. PA also can occur after dynamic testing (corticotropin releasing hormone [CRH], insulin tolerance test, thyrotropin releasing hormone [TRH] or growth hormone releasing hormone [GHRH]). Anticoagulation therapy, bleeding disorders, medications such as dopamine agonists and high-dose estrogen, radiation therapy, pregnancy, and head trauma also seem to be able to precipitate apoplexy.

PATHOPHYSIOLOGY

Apoplexy usually occurs in patients with macroadenomas. Pituitary adenomas are particularly prone to bleeding and necrosis, possibly because they outgrow their blood supply or because tumor expansion causes ischemia (and thus infarction) by compressing infundibular or superior pituitary vessels against the sellar diaphragm. The inherent fragility of tumor blood vessels may also explain the tendency to hemorrhage. Whatever the mechanism, the increase in intrasellar pressure[10,17] responsible for the swelling of neighboring structures may be more or less pronounced, explaining why the clinical spectrum ranges from "classic" acute PA to totally silent necrotic and/or hemorrhagic adenomas found on pathologic examination.

CLINICAL PRESENTATION
Headache

Headache is present in more than 80% of patients[18,19] and is generally the initial manifestation, with sudden and severe onset. It is probably due to dural traction or to extravasation of blood and necrotic material into the subarachnoid space, irritating the meninges.

Visual Disorders

Visual disorders are present at presentation in more than half of patients with PA.[3,10,18,20] They are due to a sudden hemorrhage/necrosis-related increase in tumor mass, compressing surrounding structures (mainly the optic chiasm or optic nerves, due to upward expansion of the tumor). Variable degrees of visual-field impairment may be observed, but loss of visual acuity and blindness are rare.[3,7,8,10,18]

More than half of patients with PA have ocular palsy,[21] due to functional impairment of cranial nerves III (the most affected), IV, and VI. This may be related to intracavernous expansion of the tumor mass, to a hematoma, or, most probably, to an abrupt pressure increase in the pituitary region.

Other Neurologic Signs

Signs and symptoms of meningeal irritation, such as photophobia, nausea, vomiting, meningismus, and sometimes fever, may be misleading. Consciousness may be altered, with lethargy, stupor, or even coma. Cerebral ischemia can occasionally result from mechanical compression of the carotid artery against the anterior clinoid, or cerebral vasospasm, leading to focal neurologic deficits, such as hemiparesis and dysphasia, or to a pyramidal syndrome.[22,23]

Proposed Scoring System

The UK Pituitary Apoplexy Guidelines Development Group proposed a "PA score" to quantify neuro-ophthalmic defects, based on the level of consciousness, visual acuity and field defects, and ocular palsies.[20]

ENDOCRINE DYSFUNCTION

Acute endocrine dysfunction also may be present, complicating the clinical picture. At least one anterior pituitary deficiency is always present at PA onset.[3,4,6,7,9,20,24,25] In retrospect, it is often realized that signs and symptoms of endocrine abnormalities were present before the apoplectic episode (eg, sexual problems, menstrual disturbances, galactorrhea, fatigue). These disorders are due to a mass effect on the normal pituitary.

Corticotropic Deficiency

Corticotropic deficiency is the most common deficit in patients with PA, affecting 60% to 80% of patients. It is also the most life-threatening hormonal complication, potentially causing severe hemodynamic disorders and hyponatremia. Empirical steroid supplementation should be offered to all patients with signs of PA, without waiting for diagnostic confirmation.

Other Pituitary Hormone Deficiencies

Other pituitary defects do not raise the same degree of concern in the acute setting. According to reviews of the literature,[10,25] respectively 40% to 50% and 75% to 85% of patients with PA have thyrotropic and gonadotropic deficiency at presentation. Apoplexy is one of the rare circumstances in which a pituitary adenoma may be associated with low prolactin levels[20,25] or with diabetes insipidus.

DIAGNOSIS

Diagnosis relies on a combination of clinical manifestations (eg, headaches and visual disturbances) and the presence of a pituitary adenoma, whether previously known or discovered during the workup. Imaging studies are thus crucial for diagnosis.

Computed Tomography

Computed tomography (CT) is the initial emergency examination of choice for patients who present with severe headache of sudden onset suggestive of subarachnoid hemorrhage. CT can help to eliminate this diagnosis by showing an intrasellar mass (Fig. 1), with hemorrhagic components in 80% of cases. CT is most useful in the acute setting (24–48 hours); after this time, blood intensity decreases and may be difficult to detect. After administration of contrast medium, the pituitary appears hyperdense and inhomogeneous,[26] sometimes with ring enhancement or a high-intensity fluid level.

Magnetic Resonance Imaging

MRI can identify hemorrhagic areas and show the relationship between the tumor and neighboring structures, such as the optic chiasm, cavernous sinuses, and

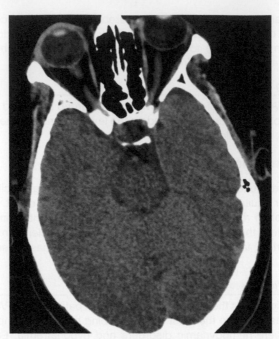

Fig. 1. CT scan at the onset of apoplexy showing a hypodense area in the adenoma reflecting intrapituitary necrosis.

hypothalamus.[27] MRI is the best means of identifying blood components in the subacute setting (4 days–1 month). It cannot replace CT in the acute setting, as it is unable to detect fresh blood.[26] MRI can show clear signal changes on T1-weighted and T2-weighted sequences, depending on the type of blood component (**Table 1**).[28]

Table 1 Blood component density changes with time on CT and MRI		
	Hemorrhage	**Necrosis**
A: CT		
Acute (0–10 d)	Hyperdensity (60–80 HU)	Hypodensity
Subacute (10–20 d)	Isodensity (40 HU)	
Chronic (>20 d)	Hypodensity (10 HU)	
B: MRI		
Acute		Hypo T1, Hyper T2
Oxyhemoglobin (<24 h)	Iso T1, Iso T2	
Deoxyhemoglobin (24–48 h)	Iso T1, Hypo T2	
Subacute		
Intracellular methemoglobin (3–5 d)	Hyper T1, Hypo T2	
Extracellular methemoglobin (>5 d)	Hyper T1, Hyper T2	
Chronic		
Hemosiderin (>3 wk)	Hypo T1, Hypo T2	

Abbreviations: CT, computed tomography; Hyper, hyperintense; Hypo, hypointense; Iso, isointense.
From Chanson P, Lepeintre JF, Ducreux D. Management of pituitary apoplexy. Expert Opin Pharmacother 2004;5:1287–98; with permission.

T1-weighted MRI can provide evidence of a pituitary lesion with intralesional areas of high signal intensity suggesting the presence of blood, and/or low intensity suggesting the presence of necrosis (**Fig. 2**). Sometimes the entire lesion can exhibit high signal intensity or a fluid-filled space, possibly associated with a fluid level inside the pituitary lesion (**Fig. 3**). In this case, the upper compartment appears hyperintense and the lower compartment isointense.

T2-weighted images show areas of both low and high signal intensity (see **Fig. 2**). A special sequence, T2*-weighted gradient-echo MRI, is able to detect intratumoral hemorrhage in pituitary adenomas with various dark aspects ("rim," "mass," "spot," "diffuse"), combinations of which could be useful for the assessment of recent and old intratumoral hemorrhagic events.[29]

Thickening of the sphenoid sinus mucosa, especially in the compartment just beneath the sella turcica, was first observed by Arita and colleagues[30] on MRI performed during the acute stage of PA. A histologic study showed that the subepithelial layer of the sphenoid sinus mucous membrane was markedly swollen.

DIFFERENTIAL DIAGNOSIS

The clinical presentation of PA may raise 2 differential diagnoses, namely subarachnoid hemorrhage and bacterial meningitis. Lumbar puncture is of little help in differentiating subarachnoid hemorrhage and bacterial meningitis from PA, as the latter may be accompanied by a high red cell count, xanthochromia or pleocytosis, and an increased cerebrospinal fluid (CSF) protein level, particularly when meningeal irritation is present. However, CSF culture will rule out bacterial meningitis, and lumbar puncture is thus mandatory if this diagnostic possibility is raised.

MANAGEMENT OF PITUITARY APOPLEXY
A Matter of Debate

Owing to the highly variable course of PA and to the limited experience of individual physicians, the optimal management of acute episodes remains controversial. At all events, PA needs to be managed by an expert multidisciplinary team, including ophthalmologists, neuroradiologists, endocrinologists, and, obviously, neurosurgeons.[20] The treatment aims are to improve symptoms and relieve compression of local structures, particularly the optic pathways. Surgical decompression is probably the most rapid means of achieving these goals. The dramatic picture presented by many patients probably explains why PA is considered a neurosurgical emergency and was almost always treated surgically in the past. However, surgery carries a risk of CSF rhinorrhea, damage to the posterior pituitary (risk of permanent diabetes insipidus) and hypopituitarism due to removal of normal pituitary tissue. The incidence of these complications falls with the experience of the neurosurgeon.

Steroid Therapy is Mandatory in Pituitary Apoplexy

As corticotropic deficiency is present in the vast majority of patients and may be life-threatening, whether PA is treated surgically or conservatively, intravenous corticosteroids must be administered immediately, even before possible surgical decompression: this treatment will consist of hydrocortisone 50 mg every 6 hours,[10,31] or a bolus of 100 to 200 mg followed by 50 to 100 mg every 6 hours intravenously (or intramuscularly), or 2 to 4 mg per hour by continuous intravenous administration.[20]

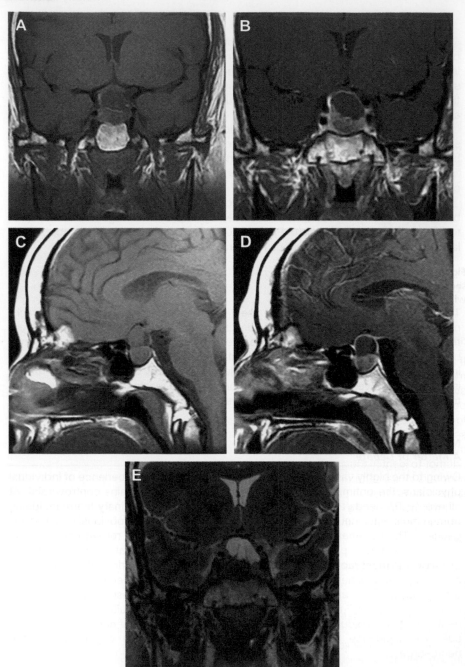

Fig. 2. MRI in the same patient as in **Fig. 1,** with symptomatic PA. The lesion is globally hypointense in T1-weighted sequences (*A*), coronal section; (*B*), sagittal section, before gadolinium injection, the upper part of the lesion being more hypointense (suggesting necrosis) than the lower part, corresponding to the solid part of the adenoma. This is confirmed by injection of gadolinium, which enhanced the signal of the solid part of the adenoma, whereas the upper part of the lesion (necrotic) remains hypointense, both on coronal (*C*) and sagittal (*D*) sections. On T2-weighted sequence, coronal section (*E*), the necrotic part of the lesion appears hyperintense.

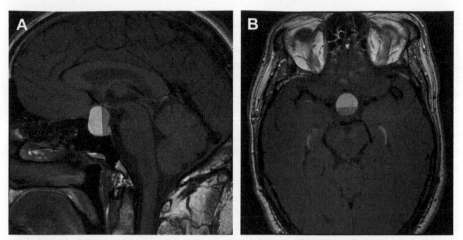

Fig. 3. MRI T1-weighted sequences, sagittal (A) and axial (B) views in a patient with a PA, showing a fluid level inside the pituitary lesion, the upper compartment being hyperintense whereas the lower is isointense.

Surgical Approach

If a surgical option is chosen, the transphenoidal approach is almost always recommended because it allows good decompression of the optic pathways and neuroanatomic structures in contact with the tumor and because it is associated with low postoperative morbidity and mortality.[20] Transphenoidal surgery is now usually performed by transnasal septal displacement rather than by the classic sublabial transeptal approach. Most neurosurgeons now prefer an endoscope to an operative microscope. The goal being optical pathway decompression, the surgeon must attempt to identify the sellar diaphragm. Gross subtotal removal is preferred if the adenoma is invasive. Endocrine outcome after elective pituitary surgery is poorer in patients with PA than in patients with nonapoplectic adenomas.[5]

In this acute setting, the operation sometimes has to be performed by an on-call neurosurgeon rather than by a skilled pituitary neurosurgeon, as underlined in UK guidelines.[20]

Conservative Approach

Reports of spontaneous clinical improvement and shrinkage (or disappearance) of apoplectic pituitary adenomas suggest that a conservative approach may be appropriate in selected cases. Pelkonen and colleagues[32] were among the first to propose a conservative approach, after observing not only spontaneous recoveries but also cases in which the PA appeared to cure hormonal hypersecretion (eg, growth hormone, adrenocorticotropic hormone). In 1995, Maccagnan and colleagues[33] reported the results of a prospective study in which they treated PA with high-dose steroids. Only patients whose visual impairment or altered consciousness failed to improve underwent surgery. Conservative steroid treatment was possible in 7 of 12 patients, leaving only 5 patients who needed surgery. Visual defects resolved in 6 of the 7 patients and improved in the remaining patient. Importantly, the posttreatment prevalence of pituitary hormone deficiency and the incidence of tumor regrowth were similar in conservatively and surgically treated patients.

Surgery or Conservative Management?

Three large retrospective studies have compared the outcomes of conservatively and surgically treated patients with PA.[6,9,24] As their investigators acknowledged, these studies suffered from a selection bias due to their retrospective design: indeed, patients in the conservative group generally had less-severe ocular defects than those in the surgical group.[10,20] This has been confirmed in a recent study[11] in which retrospective calculation of the PA score (PAS, see previously)[20] was made showing that patients treated with early surgery had lower PAS than those treated conservatively. Nevertheless, as detailed later in this article, when comparing the outcomes of PA according to the type of management in these 3 studies, results were more or less similar.[34]

Oculomotor palsies resolved completely in 64% to 100% of patients managed conservatively and in 63% to 75% of patients with surgery.[6,9,24]

Visual outcome is poorer in patients with severe disorders, such as monocular or binocular blindness, irrespective of the choice of conservative or surgical management.[8,24,35] However, the rates of visual acuity and visual-field recovery or improvement are similar after conservative and surgical treatment: visual acuity normalized in 45% to 75% of patients and improved in 25% to 36% in studies comparing the 2 strategies,[6,9,24] whereas visual field defects normalized in 50% to 100% of cases and improved in 25%. Even blindness was found to resolve at the same rate (~50%) in patients treated with conservative and surgical approaches in one study,[24] in which patients with contraindications to surgery (anesthetic risk) were treated with steroids alone. Similar visual improvement also was found in a more recent study.[36]

After surgery, pituitary function recovers partially or completely in more than 50% of cases.[3,10,37] The proportions of patients with posttreatment hypocortisolism, hypothyroidism, and hypogonadism are roughly the same in the surgical and conservative groups.[6,9,24]

Another major argument in favor of the surgical approach is that surgery can remove the pituitary tumor. However, many patients have no visible tumor remnant after an apoplectic episode managed conservatively. Recently, a long-term follow-up study showed a recurrence rate of 11.1% an average of 6.6 years after surgery.[38] In a comparative study, the incidence of tumor regrowth was low (<5%) and similar with the 2 approaches,[6] whereas it was higher after surgery in another study (22% vs 0% with conservative treatment)[24]; only 1 of these 3 comparative studies suggested that surgery was associated with a lower rate of tumor regrowth (4% vs 22% after conservative treatment).[9] Likewise, Leyer and colleagues[36] found that tumor regrowth occurred only in the conservative treatment group (17% vs 0%). Thus, the respective merits of the 2 approaches in terms of tumor control are currently difficult to judge.

United Kingdom Guidelines for the Management of Pituitary Apoplexy

Guidelines were recently proposed in the United Kingdom for the management of patients with PA.[20] Surgical decompression is recommended in case of "significant neuro-ophthalmic signs or a reduced level of consciousness." This seems a very reasonable option. If surgery is chosen, then its timing is important. It used to be believed that visual defects were a neurosurgical emergency. In fact, outcome is the same if surgery is performed during the first 3 days or the first week after PA onset.[8] Nevertheless, if the patient is operated on more than 1 week after onset, then the prognosis of any visual defects is less good: in one study, 86% of visual disorders improved or resolved when surgery took place within 8 days, versus 46% between 9 and 34 days.[3]

SUMMARY

PA, a rare clinical syndrome caused by sudden hemorrhaging or infarction of the pituitary gland, generally within a pituitary adenoma, can be difficult to diagnose. A CT or MRI scan confirms the diagnosis by revealing a pituitary tumor with hemorrhagic and/or necrotic components. Corticotropic deficiency may be life-threatening if left untreated, and glucocorticoid treatment must therefore always be initiated immediately. Owing to the highly variable outcome of this syndrome and the absence of randomized prospective studies, optimal management of acute PA is controversial. Some investigators advocate early transphenoidal surgical decompression for all patients, whereas others adopt a conservative approach for selected patients (those without visual acuity or field defects and with normal consciousness). Reevaluation of pituitary function and the tumor mass in the months following the acute apoplectic episode is mandatory to determine whether or not the pituitary defect is permanent, to check the potential hypersecretory pattern of the adenoma, and to initiate follow-up of a possible tumor remnant.

REFERENCES

1. Fernandez A, Karavitaki N, Wass JA. Prevalence of pituitary adenomas: a community-based, cross-sectional study in Banbury (Oxfordshire, UK). Clin Endocrinol (Oxf) 2010;72:377–82.
2. Raappana A, Koivukangas J, Ebeling T, et al. Incidence of pituitary adenomas in Northern Finland in 1992-2007. J Clin Endocrinol Metab 2010;95:4268–75.
3. Randeva HS, Schoebel J, Byrne J, et al. Classical pituitary apoplexy: clinical features, management and outcome. Clin Endocrinol (Oxf) 1999;51:181–8.
4. Dubuisson AS, Beckers A, Stevenaert A. Classical pituitary tumour apoplexy: clinical features, management and outcomes in a series of 24 patients. Clin Neurol Neurosurg 2007;109:63–70.
5. Moller-Goede DL, Brandle M, Landau K, et al. Pituitary apoplexy: re-evaluation of risk factors for bleeding into pituitary adenomas and impact on outcome. Eur J Endocrinol 2011;164:37–43.
6. Ayuk J, McGregor EJ, Mitchell RD, et al. Acute management of pituitary apoplexy– surgery or conservative management? Clin Endocrinol (Oxf) 2004;61:747–52.
7. Semple PL, Webb MK, de Villiers JC, et al. Pituitary apoplexy. Neurosurgery 2005;56:65–72 [discussion: 73].
8. Turgut M, Ozsunar Y, Basak S, et al. Pituitary apoplexy: an overview of 186 cases published during the last century. Acta Neurochir (Wien) 2010;152:749–61.
9. Sibal L, Ball SG, Connolly V, et al. Pituitary apoplexy: a review of clinical presentation, management and outcome in 45 cases. Pituitary 2004;7:157–63.
10. Nawar RN, AbdelMannan D, Selman WR, et al. Pituitary tumor apoplexy: a review. J Intensive Care Med 2008;23:75–90.
11. Bujawansa S, Thondam SK, Steele C, et al. Presentation, management and outcomes in acute pituitary apoplexy: a large single-centre experience from the United Kingdom. Clin Endocrinol (Oxf) 2014;80:419–24.
12. Fernandez-Balsells MM, Murad MH, Barwise A, et al. Natural history of nonfunctioning pituitary adenomas and incidentalomas: a systematic review and metaanalysis. J Clin Endocrinol Metab 2011;96:905–12.
13. Sivakumar W, Chamoun R, Nguyen V, et al. Incidental pituitary adenomas. Neurosurg Focus 2011;31:E18.
14. Biousse V, Newman NJ, Oyesiku NM. Precipitating factors in pituitary apoplexy. J Neurol Neurosurg Psychiatr 2001;71:542–5.

15. Semple PL, Jane JA Jr, Laws ER Jr. Clinical relevance of precipitating factors in pituitary apoplexy. Neurosurgery 2007;61:956–61 [discussion: 961–2].

16. Chang CV, Araujo RV, Nunes VD, et al. Predisposing factors for pituitary apoplexy. In: Turgut M, Mahapatra AK, Powell M, et al, editors. Pituitary apoplexy. Berlin: Springer-Verlag; 2014. p. 21–4.

17. Zayour DH, Selman WR, Arafah BM. Extreme elevation of intrasellar pressure in patients with pituitary tumor apoplexy: relation to pituitary function. J Clin Endocrinol Metab 2004;89:5649–54.

18. Russel SJ, Miller KK. Pituitary apoplexy. In: Swearingen B, Biller BM, editors. Diagnosis and management of pituitary disorders. Totowa (NJ): Humana Press; 2008. p. 353–75.

19. Shimon I. Clinical features of pituitary apoplexy. In: Turgut M, Mahapatra AK, Powell M, et al, editors. Pituitary apoplexy. Berlin: Springer-Verlag; 2014. p. 49–54.

20. Rajasekaran S, Vanderpump M, Baldeweg S, et al. UK guidelines for the management of pituitary apoplexy. Clin Endocrinol (Oxf) 2011;74:9–20.

21. Jenkins TM, Toosy AT. Visual acuity, eye movements and visual fields. In: Turgut M, Mahapatra AK, Powell M, et al, editors. Pituitary apoplexy. Berlin: Springer-Verlag; 2014. p. 75–88.

22. Ahmed SK, Semple PL. Cerebral ischaemia in pituitary apoplexy. Acta Neurochir (Wien) 2008;150:1193–6 [discussion: 6].

23. Mohindra S. Cerebral ischaemia in pituitary apoplexy. In: Turgut M, Mahapatra AK, Powell M, et al, editors. Pituitary apoplexy. Berlin: Springer-Verlag; 2014. p. 69–72.

24. Gruber A, Clayton J, Kumar S, et al. Pituitary apoplexy: retrospective review of 30 patients–is surgical intervention always necessary? Br J Neurosurg 2006;20:379–85.

25. Semple PL, Ross IL. Endocrinopathies and other biochemical abnormalities in pituitary apoplexy. In: Turgut M, Mahapatra AK, Powell M, et al, editors. Pituitary apoplexy. Berlin: Springer-Verlag; 2014. p. 107–15.

26. L'Huillier F, Combes C, Martin N, et al. MRI in the diagnosis of so-called pituitary apoplexy: seven cases. J Neuroradiol 1989;16:221–37 [in English, French].

27. Piotin M, Tampieri D, Rufenacht DA, et al. The various MRI patterns of pituitary apoplexy. Eur Radiol 1999;9:918–23.

28. Flanagan EP, Hunderfund AL, Giannini C, et al. Addition of magnetic resonance imaging to computed tomography and sensitivity to blood in pituitary apoplexy. Arch Neurol 2011;68:1336–7.

29. Tosaka M, Sato N, Hirato J, et al. Assessment of hemorrhage in pituitary macroadenoma by T2*-weighted gradient-echo MR imaging. AJNR Am J Neuroradiol 2007;28:2023–9.

30. Arita K, Kurisu K, Tominaga A, et al. Thickening of sphenoid sinus mucosa during the acute stage of pituitary apoplexy. J Neurosurg 2001;95:897–901.

31. Chanson P, Lepeintre JF, Ducreux D. Management of pituitary apoplexy. Expert Opin Pharmacother 2004;5:1287–98.

32. Pelkonen R, Kuusisto A, Salmi J, et al. Pituitary function after pituitary apoplexy. Am J Med 1978;65:773–8.

33. Maccagnan P, Macedo CL, Kayath MJ, et al. Conservative management of pituitary apoplexy: a prospective study. J Clin Endocrinol Metab 1995;80:2190–7.

34. Chanson P, Salenave S. Conservative management of pituitary apoplexy. In: Turgut M, Mahapatra AK, Powell M, et al, editors. Pituitary apoplexy. Berlin: Springer-Verlag; 2014. p. 151–6.

35. Muthukumar N, Rossette D, Soundaram M, et al. Blindness following pituitary apoplexy: timing of surgery and neuro-ophthalmic outcome. J Clin Neurosci 2008;15:873–9.

36. Leyer C, Castinetti F, Morange I, et al. A conservative management is preferable in milder forms of pituitary tumor apoplexy. J Endocrinol Invest 2011;34:502–9.
37. Arafah BM, Harrington JF, Madhoun ZT, et al. Improvement of pituitary function after surgical decompression for pituitary tumor apoplexy. J Clin Endocrinol Metab 1990;71:323–8.
38. Pal A, Capatina C, Tenreiro AP, et al. Pituitary apoplexy in non-functioning pituitary adenomas: long term follow up is important because of significant numbers of tumour recurrences. Clin Endocrinol (Oxf) 2011;75:501–4.

Index

Note: Page numbers of article titles are in **boldface** type.

A

Abdominal fat, effect on GH assays, 28
Acromegaly, with pituitary tumors, bone health and, 173–175
 cabergoline for, cardiac valvulopathy and, 93–94
 diagnosis of, immunoassays for, 28–29, 31, 35
  OGTT test for, 29, 35
 FIPA and, 21
 pharmacotherapy for, **35–41**
  clinical trials on, 36–39
  clinically approved agents in, 36, 40
  combination therapy in, 36, 40
  key points of, 35
  literature review on, 35
  recommendations for, 40
  resistance to, 36
  summary of, 40
 pituitary tumor phenotypes associated with, 2
 pregnancy and, 183, 187–191
  follow-up after delivery, 191
  lactation and, 190–191
  SA safety and outcomes, 187–190
  SA vs. DA efficacy, 187, 190
  summary of, 183, 187
  surgery for, 187, 190
  treatment of, 187–191
 QoL with, 164–165
  characteristic trends of, 164
  introduction to, 161–162
  multifactorial mechanisms of, 164–165
  questionnaires for, 162, 164
   results review of, 164–165
  summary of, 165
  treatment effect on, 164–165
 remission of, following endoscopic transsphenoidal pituitary surgery, 108–110
  following pituitary irradiation, 118–119
 silent GH tumor with, 82
 silent GH tumor without, 14–15
 treatment of choice for, 36, 108, 118
ACTH. See *Adrenocorticotrophic hormone (ACTH).*
ACTH modulators, for Cushing disease, in clinical practice, 52–54
 in combination therapy, 63–68
 study designs and results of, 56–58

Endocrinol Metab Clin N Am 44 (2015) 211–242
http://dx.doi.org/10.1016/S0889-8529(14)00130-3
0889-8529/15/$ – see front matter © 2015 Elsevier Inc. All rights reserved.

endo.theclinics.com

Moving?

Make sure your subscription moves with you!

To notify us of your new address, find your **Clinics Account Number** (located on your mailing label above your name), and contact customer service at:

Email: journalscustomerservice-usa@elsevier.com

800-654-2452 (subscribers in the U.S. & Canada)
314-447-8871 (subscribers outside of the U.S. & Canada)

Fax number: 314-447-8029

Elsevier Health Sciences Division
Subscription Customer Service
3251 Riverport Lane
Maryland Heights, MO 63043

*To ensure uninterrupted delivery of your subscription, please notify us at least 4 weeks in advance of move.

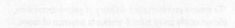

Printed and bound by CPI Group (UK) Ltd, Croydon, CR0 4YY

03/10/2024

01040485-0009